MISCARRIAGE HEARTBREAK

A FAMILY'S GUIDE TO PROCESS GRIEF, RESTORE
EMOTIONAL STRENGTH, AND LEARN EFFECTIVE
WAYS TO OFFER GENUINE SUPPORT AFTER
PREGNANCY LOSS

TAE SIMEON

CONTENTS

Introduction   5

1. Understanding Miscarriage and Its Impact   9
2. The Grieving Process: Embracing and
   Processing Loss   22
3. Physical Recovery: Caring for Your Body
   After Loss   42
4. Building Support Systems: Finding and
   Offering Help   57
5. Addressing Common Concerns and Questions   82
6. Managing Relationships After Loss   108
7. Embracing Hope and Moving Forward   123
8. It Gets Better from This Point On   135

Conclusion   143
References   147

INTRODUCTION

Let's begin with a trigger warning. I remember the day with stark clarity. I was walking around the house doing light household chores when I felt some warm fluid trickle out of me. I rushed to the bathroom to find that there were drops of blood that had come out. I tried not to panic, as I did not want to think negatively about my pregnancy. My husband asked me to accompany him to the store to grab some odds and ends, so we went. As I walked up and down the aisles, I began to feel slight cramping and even warmer fluid being expelled. I could no longer ignore what was happening. We paid for our purchase and made it back home. My attempt to remain calm went out the window immediately as I walked into my bathroom. My heart pounded in anticipation. I stood in front of the toilet and slowly removed my undergarments to find a devastating amount of blood and tissue. At that moment, my world shifted. An ER visit had confirmed what I already knew. I had just miscarried twins during my 8th week of pregnancy. Hello heartbreak. The joy and dreams I had carried were replaced with disbelief and sorrow. The feeling of isolation was immediate. I felt alone even though I was home with my family. This book is born from that moment and the journey that followed.

Fast forward to months later, as my life continued to unravel. The decision to try for another baby was not made lightly. My husband and I weighed the pros and cons of another pregnancy for months before we decided to expand our family. After all, I was just over 40 years old, so that biological clock was ticking away as if it were on a megaphone. I convinced myself that since I was of average weight, a non-smoker, non-drinker, and in general good health, I should be able to have a healthy pregnancy. And there was no way I would have back-to-back miscarriages given those characteristics, right? No ma'am. Almost a year to the day following my first miscarriage of twins, I found myself at an 8-week OBGYN appointment where the medical professionals told me that, while yes, I was pregnant again, there was no heartbeat. How could this be? That was supposed to be my Rainbow Baby! Devastation, anger, confusion, betrayal, sadness, all the somber emotions that a human can experience hit me from head to toe like an inexperienced mixed martial arts fighter taking blows from the reigning champion. Unlike the previous miscarriage, my body did not want to let go of this pregnancy. I had to endure a medical procedure under anesthesia at the main hospital to have everything inside my uterus removed. After all that was over, I was left with three Angel babies.

Now that I have shared my personal experience with miscarriage, let's get into why you are here. You or someone you know may have had the misfortune of going through a similar encounter. This book can help guide you through this frantic time. It seeks to provide a path to emotional healing and practical support for women who have experienced miscarriage. It is also a guide for partners who are at a loss and eager to support, but unsure how. This resource is both informative and deeply empathetic. It is a companion for those managing the blustery periods of grief and recovery.

You, dear reader, are the heart of this book. Whether you are a fellow miscarriage survivor who has faced this loss herself, a partner standing by her side, or a family member wanting to understand, this book is for you. Each page is crafted with your journey in mind.

What will you gain from this book? You will learn to process the complex emotions of grief. You will discover the medical aspects of miscarriage, equipping yourself with knowledge that can empower and inform. Additionally, you will find strategies for emotional and physical recovery and realistic ways to offer genuine support. This book takes a holistic approach. It acknowledges that healing is physical, emotional, and relational.

Why is this book even necessary? Well, we must break the silence surrounding miscarriage. For too long, it has been shrouded in societal stigma. Many women suffer in silence, feeling alone in their grief. It's estimated that up to 20% of known pregnancies result in miscarriage (Mayo Clinic, n.d.). Even given that, silence persists. These figures highlight how widespread this phenomenon is, helping diminish feelings of isolation and encouraging connectivity among those affected. This universal nature patterns a painful equality, a community meshed with experiences rather than spoken words. Silence can be a barrier to healing, compounding the emotional toll. It is time for open conversations and shared stories.

This book includes diverse perspectives. You will read personal stories about me and other women and men. Stories from various cultural backgrounds offer a broad view of miscarriage experiences. These stories are a testament to resilience and the communal human experience of loss and recovery.

The book's structure is designed to guide you through this tour of newfound unfamiliarity. It begins by explaining the medical and emotional aspects of miscarriage. From there, it moves to emotional healing, offering strategies and insights to help you navigate your feelings. The next section focuses on physical recovery, providing practical advice for caring for your body. Finally, the book addresses rebuilding relationships, recognizing the impact of miscarriage on partners and families.

I invite you to engage with this book as a companion on your quest to find healing. It offers optimism and support at every step. You are not alone, and I will reinforce that message as a gentle reminder. We will move along this winding road to find strength and comfort in familiar stories and collective wisdom. Healing is a mighty undertaking, and this book is here to be with you.

CHAPTER 1
UNDERSTANDING MISCARRIAGE AND ITS IMPACT

UNDERSTANDING miscarriage and its impact transcends medical facts. It delves into emotional spaces that each of us must face and comprehend. As we unpack its complexities, a figurative boiling pot of hefty emotions, medical realities, and societal perceptions flare out before us, demanding not just understanding, but empathy and support. Miscarriage can affect women in all parts of the world, and it doesn't discriminate when it comes to victim selection. The abrupt ending of a pregnancy creates emotional wounds that could take years to mend. The impact of a miscarriage will vary from person to person, and there is no right or wrong way to move forward during the aftermath.

Grasping the full scope of miscarriage encompasses more than just an awareness of its various forms and underlying reasons. It requires profound recognition and respect for the distinctiveness of every person's journey through it. Recognizing miscarriage as common is to honor its deep personalization. This chapter frames the case for a deeper exploration into the healing pathways available on both emotional and physical levels, while dismantling mythical misconceptions that obscure clarity and compassion.

DEFINING MISCARRIAGE: TYPES AND CAUSES

In clinical terms, a miscarriage is the loss of a pregnancy before the 20th week of gestation. Yet, this definition barely scratches the surface of its diversity. Experiencing a miscarriage is not merely a physical ordeal, but one enveloped in emotional turbulence and layered narratives. There are various types, each marked by distinctive causes and manifestations. A threatened miscarriage is characterized by vaginal bleeding without cervical dilation, indicating risk rather than certainty of loss. An incomplete miscarriage, where some pregnancy tissue remains post-loss, often requires medical intervention. Conversely, a missed or silent miscarriage might proceed without symptoms. An ultrasound revealing an absent fetal heartbeat typically unveils its tragic discovery.

Ectopic pregnancies add a dimension of challenge. Here, a fertilized egg improperly implants outside the uterus, often in a fallopian tube. These pregnancies cannot continue normally and pose significant health risks if untreated, underscored by symptoms like sharp abdominal pain and vaginal bleeding. Treatment typically involves medication or surgery to protect health and prevent complications.

Molar pregnancies, albeit rare, are critical forms of pregnancy loss. With a complete molar pregnancy, abnormal growth fills the uterus, absent of an embryo, while a partial molar pregnancy includes malformed tissue alongside an embryo. Both necessitate medical care due to the risks posed, particularly regarding future pregnancies. Blighted ovum and chemical pregnancies further illustrate early pregnancy loss phenomena. A blighted ovum occurs when a fertilized egg attaches yet fails to develop into an embryo, resulting in a loss. Chemical pregnancies signify very early miscarriages post-implantation, typically detectable through early testing.

Every miscarriage is unique, flooded with stories reflecting an array of emotional landscapes. The reasons for these losses are manifold, often rooted in varied medical circumstances. Chromosomal abnormalities, prevalent among causes, involve genetic defects impairing fetal development. Maternal health concerns, including unmanaged diabetes or thyroid issues, may increase the risk. Meanwhile, lifestyle factors like smoking cigarettes and drinking alcohol can contribute as well.

These scientific explanations unveil a network of myths warranting clarification. Activities such as exercise or sexual intercourse do not induce miscarriage. Having moderate stress levels is also not a contributor. Myths like these oppress individuals with unnecessary guilt. Having a grasp on the medical realities behind miscarriages serves not only to dispel these myths but also to facilitate emotional recovery by easing the worries carried by the affected. We will take a deeper dive into miscarriage myths shortly.

EXPLORING VARIOUS TRIGGERS OF MISCARRIAGE

Examining the breadth of triggers behind miscarriages offers insights into the multifaceted nature of this experience. Environmental factors, for instance, may play unexpected roles. Exposure to radiation or certain chemicals in closed settings can inadvertently affect pregnancy viability. Comprehending these risks brings attention to protective measures necessary for pregnant individuals, advocating for safer workplaces tailored to these needs.

Genetic testing provides further clarity on chromosomal abnormalities that may lead to miscarriage. This may be an option for you if you have a nonviable fetus that needs surgical extraction. In some cases, recurrent miscarriages prompt genetic counseling to explore potential hereditary conditions contributing to loss. This proactive approach underscores the importance of personalized healthcare in managing and interpreting recurrent pregnancy challenges.

MEDICAL INSIGHTS: WHAT HAPPENS DURING A MISCARRIAGE?

Underpinning the physical process of miscarriage is a deeply personal, often painful experience. It encompasses a domino effect of biological events signaling pregnancy cessation. The cervix begins to open, a subtle but significant shift allowing the uterus to contract, reflecting the body's intrinsic, though often uncontrollable response to expulsion. To many, it is accompanied by helplessness, as their body partakes in involuntary processes.

These uterine contractions, subsequent cervical dilation, and eventual passage of tissue are observable as vaginal bleeding and cramps. The symptoms represent physical shifts and can be emotionally unnerving. Bleeding ranges from light spotting like at the beginning of a menstrual period to more prolonged events, often with tissue or clot discharge. Each can serve as an unwelcome but necessary reminder of loss. In other words, a visceral sign of the body's effort to revert to its pre-pregnancy status.

Healthcare practitioners rely on diagnostic tools to determine miscarriage. Ultrasounds detect the presence of a fetal heartbeat, a critical pregnancy marker. Its absence typically confirms miscarriage. Blood tests offer insight by measuring hormone levels like human chorionic gonadotropin (hCG). Healthy pregnancies see rising levels, but a decrease or static measurement can suggest loss.

Several management options emerge after diagnosis, tailored to specific needs and situations. Expectant management entails allowing nature to proceed without interference, suiting situations where the body is deemed capable of self-resolution. Alternatively, medical management involves medications like misoprostol to accelerate tissue expulsion. This can be useful for those preferring to expedite and conclude this emotional challenge. Keep in mind that the side effects of taking medication to induce tissue expulsion are likely to include severe cramping and discomfort, and it may not completely rid the uterus of the embryo or fetus and placenta.

In instances where natural or medical management is unsuitable or has failed, surgical procedures such as dilation and curettage (D&C) under anesthesia offer another course. The choice, replete with considerations spanning emotional, physical, and practical dimensions, warrants thorough consultation with healthcare providers.

While grieving, the array of choices might feel overwhelming; however, decisions remain deeply personal, reflecting individual circumstances and needs. No choice is fundamentally right or wrong, as each provides a unique resolution and solace. Understanding miscarriage aids in demystifying it, empowering individuals to make informed care decisions. Your healthcare provider will explain all the options to guide you in deciding. Something must be done, so unfortunately, not deciding isn't an option.

These medical insights acknowledge strength and perseverance. The body endures exceedingly difficult things, but it still provides a course to healing and recovery. Recognizing these physiological elements informs and validates experiences, equipping individuals with the knowledge necessary to cover this vast terrain.

Actionable Item: Understanding Your Options

Ponder the physiological process of miscarriage and management choices. Consider how this aligns with your experience or concerns. If you have already experienced a miscarriage, did you require medical intervention? Do you know what type of miscarriage you had? If chromosomal testing were made available, would you opt in and receive results? Record questions or reflections regarding how you would approach these decisions upon facing them anew or for the first time.

COMMON MISCONCEPTIONS AND MYTHS

Encapsulated within miscarriage are misconceptions, further compounding its emotional load. A prevailing myth is its supposed preventability. It supposes that, with care, miscarriage might be circumvented. Reality defies this notion. Health practices contribute to healthier pregnancies, but many miscarriages stem from uncontrollable factors, like chromosomal anomalies. Such genetic irregularities defy premeditation or prevention. This misconception breeds unfounded guilt, misplacing a sense of culpability after loss.

Another enduring myth presupposes miscarriage as a harbinger of fertility concerns. It suggests a notion that future conceivability is compromised, fueling undue apprehension for those aspiring to conceive again. In truth, most women who have had a miscarriage achieve successful subsequent pregnancies, especially with time and guidance. Dispelling this myth is of the essence, for it propagates unnecessary anxiety divorced from factual foundations. Medical evidence offers a contrasting optic, affirming that miscarriage, though common, does not inherently indicate continued reproductive impediments. The medical community champions the inclination that success following a miscarriage is not only possible but likely. This line of thinking dispels tormenting myths that spurn distress and misinformation.

Everyday stress, exercise, lifting moderately heavy objects, previously taking birth control, or even drinking soda or a cup of coffee are all common daily aspects of life, yet they contribute to miscarriage myths. None of these factors has been proven to cause miscarriage. Additionally, the misconception that pregnancy loss only happens during the early stages is false. While the textbook definition of miscarriage marks the end of a pregnancy within the first 20 weeks, fetal development can cease at any point during the nine months of pregnancy.

One of the most harmful misconceptions is when people tell others not to grieve because they don't think the baby was even real yet. Misconceptions such as these wield a poignant influence on emotional wellness. They foment self-doubt and perceive inadequacy. Picture a woman inwardly absorbing a myth-laden narrative that miscarriage equates to maternal deficiency. This accusation forms layered grief, which is unjustly clouded by potential fallibility. Misconceptions resonate beyond the individual, often influencing partners and family intimately.

STRATEGIES TO COMBAT MISCONCEPTIONS

Advocating educational outreach remains crucial in combating persistent myths. Healthcare professionals are pivotal in disseminating accurate information and debunking fallacies shrouded in misinterpretation. National campaigns raising awareness and dispelling myths could transform public reasoning, engendering an informed community advocating for truth over tradition.

Fight back against misconceptions by leading with facts, not fear. For example, when someone verbalizes a myth that working out will cause a miscarriage, let them know that most exercise is safe for mom and baby and encouraged, until a doctor says otherwise. Reference credible sources like well-known medical journals or organizations to support your claims.

It's important to actively spread accurate information and debunk these myths for emotional well-being. Sharing educational information and upholding open dialogue based on reality guards against stereotypes. Having factual conversations and encouraging dialogue fortified by truth diminishes taboos, replacing avoidance with understanding.

Let's envision a scenario at a community event where one individual's courage promotes conversation, sharing their miscarriage testimony. That bravery prompts fellow attendees to cast aside secrecy to voice their stories, provoking a chain reaction where benevolence and support thrive. Collective enlightenment chips away at long-held myths to bolster inclusive interpretation.

Addressing myths directly not only bolsters personal healing but also endorses a culture of honesty where miscarriage is discussed candidly. By embracing accuracy and engaging with inclusive dialogue, we lessen the disconnection surrounding those impacted by miscarriage. This myth-busting crusade hinges upon education and advocacy, dismantling antiquated lore for informed conversations. Healthcare involvement ensures authenticity, coupling evidence with empathy to extend practice-informed support.

Solidarity amplifies impact in countering these tenacious myths. Each dialogue and declared account contributes to an expanding community full of knowledge and care capable of transforming the societal lens on miscarriage. The ripple effects incited are felt beyond individual healing as they contribute to a significant momentum toward societal acceptance and comprehensive support, forging a new legacy grounded in truth and compassion.

THE EMOTIONAL TOLL: DEALING WITH THE IMMEDIATE AFTERMATH

Following a miscarriage, emotions frequently surge and bombard your spirit with an unsavory fervor of all kinds of feelings. Shock often presides with a numbing disbelief, muting any sense of reality. It is common to feel ensnared in a surreal storyline, hoping for an awakening that restores normality. Yet as reality announces itself, extreme grief and sadness take hold, casting a cloud over one's heart. This grief is distinct, periodically tagged with emptiness and a longing for possibilities lost.

Subtle yet pernicious guilt often sneaks in, layering doubt over actions one might have altered. These emotions, while common, are usually baseless. It is natural to seek control during chaos, but it's necessary to concede that miscarriage often evades personal control.

Identifying and employing coping strategies is imperative to address the immediate emotional turmoil effectively. Journaling serves as a vehicle for unspoken thoughts, and writing provides a cathartic space for emotional release. Equally, deep breathing techniques can mitigate anxiety. Simple exercises, like inhaling deeply and exhaling slowly, can ground one, instilling calmness.

Seeking support plays a compelling role in moving through this emotional quagmire. Though daunting, confiding in a trusted ally provides comfort. Sharing one's experience with an empathetic listener aids healing. When familial exchanges are overwhelming, professional counseling offers guided steps. Therapists specializing in grief can coach emotional exploration and provide personalized coping strategies.

Grieving assumes a deep personal nature, varying intrinsically from one to another. Some might maneuver through emotions swiftly, traversing grief stages with unexpected celerity. Others need more time, gleaning the loss's full magnitude before catching on. There is no definitive grieving timeline, only a reminder that individual experiences dictate different needs.

Consider a friend confronting a similar loss. She might immerse herself in productivity to distract and to cope. Meanwhile, another friend might necessitate withdrawal and quiet contemplation. Both methods are valid, underscoring individual variance in grieving.

Recognizing this variability suggests compassion as a noteworthy ally. Permitting oneself to grieve distinctly is fundamental. It's important to affirm that grieving does not adhere to a set pattern or societal expectations. Like a plane ride, it can be calm at one moment and turbulent the next. Accepting this fluctuation is key to the handling of grief.

THE ROLE OF SUPPORT SYSTEMS IN MITIGATING IMPACT

The availability and quality of support systems are significant factors in processing miscarriage. Partners play pivotal roles, even as they surmise their own emotions. Open communication strengthens mutual understanding, backing a supportive moral force necessary for recovery. A partner's presence and tenderness can significantly lighten an individual's load, reminding them they are not alone.

Healthcare providers also serve as vital resources, offering medical guidance and emotional support. Compassionate care from practitioners helps patients endure medical procedures with dignity and respect. This professional support is invaluable, ensuring patients receive thorough explanations of their options and potential outcomes. Such guidance often includes recommending mental health resources for additional support.

Reaching out to available resources provides security during such emotional transitions. Support groups tailored to miscarriage offer compassion-driven environments, furthering collective healing through stories. Online communities provide anonymity, often encouraging open dialogues regarding personal hardships and reflections.

Remember that there is someone who has undergone this struggle in these early days after a miscarriage. Numerous others have felt, and may feel, this painful part of life. The emotions you harbor connect you to a vast community of those who assimilate deep vulnerabilities. In this collective space, seek solace knowing that support isn't a mark of frailty. Whether leaning on close circles or accessing professional avenues, these supports serve as critical lifelines when moments turn into gloom. Accept grief for being as unique as it is pressing to provide the groundwork for healing. Foregoing pressure for preordained timelines and conceding that healing is singular to everyone develops hopefulness during grief. Despite its challenges, walking through this chapter of life underscores the resilience and determination inherent within you.

Encouraging closure and connecting with others who have encountered similar experiences can advance fellowship and diminish feelings of isolation. Online forums and support groups offer digital sanctuaries where personal stories interweave, forming a collective portrait of the spirit of toughness and commiseration. Engaging in these communities provides reassurance and validation, which is needed in the healing process. Every account is cherished and significant, incorporating medical interventions or natural resolution. Sharing these tales promotes awareness for oneself and those enduring similar challenges. Recognizing the variability of experience and commonality, we harness strength in unity.

Actionable Item: Exploring Your Experience

In reflection, pause to consider your personal encounter with miscarriage. Journaling may provide a canvas to document your experience, examining sentiments from the initial signs of loss to your current comprehension of events. What emotions did you encounter? How did your body react? Catalog the support accessible to you throughout this ordeal. Use this introspection to celebrate your story and process emotions within a haven.

CHAPTER 2
THE GRIEVING PROCESS: EMBRACING AND PROCESSING LOSS

STAGES OF GRIEF: RECOGNIZING THE WAVES OF EMOTION

THERE ARE five stages of grief: denial and shock, anger and frustration, bargaining and self-reflection, depression and deep sorrow, and acceptance and adjustment. Personal experience with these stages will vary as the stages are nonlinear. Some will revisit stages multiple times, while others may skim past one and become stuck in a different stage for a prolonged period. If I can interject for just a second, I would tell you that I revisited anger and frustration as well as depression and deep sorrow multiple times in a three-year window. I very recently moved to acceptance and adjustment.

So, you may be wondering, how long does getting through the stages of grief take, and will you ever feel normal again? Grief can be a short period of time for some and long and drawn out for others. It truly depends on the person. For me, I was done grieving after three years. Although I do have some moments of sadness here and there, I am functional now and at the point where I have accepted what has happened. Other people may be able to progress faster. You will feel normal again after you flow through all the stages of grief.

Grief has no assigned expiration and can present itself at the most inopportune times. Something as simple as going for a walk and seeing a woman push a stroller can catapult someone grieving a miscarriage into a state of depression when they were previously in denial. Humans have emotions for a reason, and we are all justified in feeling whatever we feel. The cycles of emotion can be mighty, stopping us in our tracks, or they can be gentle and calm, requiring light navigation.

JOURNALING AS A HEALING TOOL: WRITING THROUGH TEARS

An effective strategy to combat grief is journaling. This is easier to do now since almost everyone has a smartphone handy. Grab your phone and compose an email draft of exactly how you feel in the moment, regardless of whether you can only see the negatives. Eventually, you will have something positive to write about. Even if that positive thing was that you had your favorite ice cream for the first time in a long time, and for five minutes, you didn't have a care in the world. Free writing may be better suited for you on certain days, while at other times, you may want to follow structured prompts that focus on a specific thing, like emotion. Writing about gratitude may be a challenge to some at first, but it's worth trying. One sentence at a time is the way to get going.

Journaling offers a private oasis against disturbance, a hiding place where thoughts spill freely and emotions unearth their voice. This liberated form of expression, often through stream-of-consciousness writing, allows unfiltered thoughts to surface, revealing insights that might stay hidden during spoken conversations. A blank page acts as a gateway for exploration, providing clarity in times of emotional unrest.

Utilizing journal prompts can enhance your introspection. Perhaps consider reflecting on those moments when your grief felt most intense, documenting the elaborate emotions surrounding that period. Writing heartfelt letters to your unborn child that capture unsaid dreams and love provides a canvas for processing unspoken feelings. These exercises are not born from the desire to create literary masterpieces but are driven by a need to express truthfully what's nestled within. By engaging with these prompts, words can console your spirit, allowing you to reach and soothe the deeper layers of grief.

Engaging in regular writing becomes a means to capture snapshots of your emotional evolution, marking significant shifts over time. Revisiting these entries during challenging periods may decipher recurring patterns in your responses, boosting empowerment by demonstrating your progress as a testament to strength and growth.

Introducing creativity into journaling injects depth into the healing process. Incorporating poetry or meaningful quotes can transform your work into a vibrant testament to the time you spend shepherding grief. This creative interaction summons an element of lightheartedness and invites discovery, providing unexpectedly transformative healing avenues. The quiet embrace offers a sense of calm and space, enabling exploration of grief without intolerance. The sacred dialogue between you and the text becomes a haven, opening a realm where hope and healing can flourish unabated.

ACKNOWLEDGING YOUR GRIEF: IT'S OKAY TO FEEL

Time plays a huge role in grief. No one can tell you how long to grieve, or that you should be past something by a specific time. Grief is very personal, and everyone moves with it at the pace that is right for them. Time allows you to see each stage of grief and process it. We all grieve differently, and taking the time to sit with your genuine emotions can be gratifying.

In those still moments, when the world retreats into silence and self-awareness sharpens, the acute depth of grief is revealed in elaborate expressions. The sense of loss is deep and lasting, becoming a part of who you are and creating a complicated, overflowing cup of sorrow. This temporary mourning lifestyle encompasses a spectrum of emotions as a frenzied whirlwind reshapes your inner landscape. Emotions like anger, resentment, and intense unanticipated sadness erupt not as symbols of fragility but as testaments to your humanity and your vast capacity for love. These responses are natural and fundamentally ingrained aspects of being human.

Seemingly innocuous triggers can summon a deluge of grief. The timelessness of a song or the frozen moment of a photograph can evoke a torrent of emotions, abruptly reviving memories of your loss. Though these triggers can be painful, they are indispensable. They spotlight the void left by the departed, emphasizing the significance and reach of what once was part of your life. These piercing reminders can be catalysts, spearheading raw, honest emotional exchanges. Every tear is not merely a sign of vulnerability but an acknowledgment and release, a bitter step along the way to find healing.

Sailing through these waves of emotions demands bravery and a conscious act of self-kindness. It's important to embed compassion into your daily life, treating yourself as lovingly as you would a cherished friend in need. Grieving isn't about exhibiting strength, but it showcases a deeply personal experience requiring respect and realization for its distinct path. Permit yourself to experience your own emotions without the interference of worrying about how others perceive your process. This type of sensitivity becomes the bedrock of healing and guides you toward a future of grace and newfound strength.

Expressing emotions outwardly can provide immense relief. The act of confiding in someone you trust can transform grief from an isolating experience into an open dialogue. Human connection becomes a backbone during bleak times, solidifying the concept that despite the isolation grief may induce, someone is with you every step of the way. Through shared sorrow, you find support, diminishing the heaviness of grief as others help shoulder your emotional load.

Refrain from comparing your grieving process to others. Whether your grief is chaotic, overwhelming, or quietly persistent, it warrants respect and recognition. By honoring your personal process of grief and allowing emotions to reveal themselves naturally, authentic healing will emerge in its own time and form, evolving with each passing moment. Practicing patience and self-compassion transforms moments of vulnerability into grit, allowing your unique trial to unfold at its own pace, freed from arbitrary timelines.

You may find yourself asking the question: "How do I cope with the overwhelming feeling of loss?" While there is no simple answer, I can offer you what worked for me, as I did a variety of things. I started by eating my feelings as a coping mechanism. I collected as many endorphins as possible through food that tasted great, not just good. I ate all my favorites regularly. Cakes, donuts, soft serve ice cream, seafood, tacos, you name it. I needed to feel good, and food was there for me. Of course I gained twenty-five pounds in the process, but hey, I just lost my babies so it's pregnancy weight, right? I was also a huge fan of having distractions. I did whatever I could to keep myself busy because I found out through trial and error that just sitting still around the house was deepening my depression. Weird concept, I know, since I consider myself a homebody. I found myself withdrawing from almost everything and I was deep in the trenches of isolation with my tear ducts working overtime. At some point, I sought out support through a small group of friends and family. When all else failed, I joined a Facebook support group for miscarriage, and then I eventually attended weekly grief counseling sessions with two different therapists over three months. There, I learned to incorporate journaling, which I did on my phone for easy access. This process, along with time, led me to finally see that healing is possible.

Actionable Item: Self-Compassion Checklist

During this testing period, evaluate the kindness you extend to yourself. Use this checklist as a reminder to practice self-compassion daily:

- Make it a habit to speak to yourself with gentleness, using affirming language.

- Allow yourself to rest, recognizing that rest is not synonymous with guilt or inadequacy.
- Engage in comforting activities that spark even fleeting joy and serenity.
- Set achievable goals and cherish small victories.
- Proclaim and celebrate tiny steps of progress towards healing.
- Never shy away from seeking help and support; doing so exemplifies courage.

Frequently turn to this checklist as a reminder to integrate self-care into your style towards healing.

MINDFULNESS AND MEDITATION: FINDING PEACE IN THE PRESENT

Mindfulness serves as a lighthouse on the shrouded shore of loss, binding you to the present moment amid tumultuous memories of the past and concerns of the future. Focusing intently on the now allows mindfulness to invite unhindered, non-hypocritical engagement with your thoughts and feelings, encouraging acceptance without attachment, offering clarity and grace during emotional mayhem. By enhancing awareness, mindfulness urges fulfillment of each moment as it is, enabling an embrace of emotions with calm acceptance.

To hone mindfulness, foundational meditation techniques can instill relaxation and presence. Breathing exercises offer a simple method of grounding. Intentional, deep breaths synchronize the rhythm of breathing with the flow of thoughts, providing stability. Alternatively, a body scan guides awareness through each part of your physical being, diffusing tension while creating a connection to bodily sensations.

Deep breathing exercises are beneficial for activating the parasympathetic nervous system, which handles your rest and digest response. This act is excellent for lowering your blood pressure, which most likely has become elevated during this ordeal, and it can reduce stress and anxiety. You can do deep breathing exercises anywhere. Some places could be in your car, the break room at work, aisle 5 in the grocery store, or in line at your favorite deli. The locations are endless.

Mindfulness peels back the layers of grief, permitting emotions to arise and be unveiled without discernment. These emotions are perceived as temporary visitors rather than permanent fixtures, allowing for compassionate engagement. It also leads to shifts in your relationship with grief, encouraging a grounding presence that aids in embracing emotions without becoming entrenched by them. Mindfulness honors the coexistence of loss and enduring life by promoting understanding and acceptance. This practice becomes a companion for you, ensuring emotions are processed constructively rather than left lingering and festering.

Mindfulness practices hold sentinel roles in reflective healing trajectories. Integrating mindfulness embraces presence by grounding emotional upheaval while observing thoughts and emotions with forgiving kindness. This curved practice ties the bond between mind and body, recognizing the discrete, yet united impacts of emotions on physical health. Practicing mindfulness introduces resoluteness and self-compassion, integral tools in processing grief.

Fusing holistic into mainstream therapies lays fertile ground for grasping the mind and body symbiosis, recognizing that physical and emotional healing follow diverse, interconnected tracks. Integrating these practices declares that recovery incorporates emotional life's contours beyond physical remedies alone.

Resources such as mindfulness apps and literature deepen avenues to explore and decipher these transformative practices. Apps like Headspace and Calm bring structured meditations seamlessly into your everyday life, while books offer deeper insights into varied perspectives and applications.

CREATING FUTURE-FOCUSED VISUALIZATIONS

Visualizing an unwavering outlook for the future is a powerful thing you can do to transcend fear. Congratulations are in order if you find yourself thinking about future visualizations, because that means you are one step closer to finding healing. Feeling uncertain and disconnected from the future is normal after experiencing a loss. A future-focused visualization can help you to restore hope, create and maintain emotional safety, and become familiar again with things that resonate with you the most.

A step-by-step approach to this is as follows:

Step 1: Choose a calm and quiet spot as your emotional safe space to get cozy. Set the mood by lighting a candle or playing soft music, or anything else that would help you feel grounded or supported. Be mindful that this process is not about forgetting what just happened, rather it is about honoring the experience and being open to what comes next.

Step 2: Allow yourself to be fully present in the moment with no distractions. Close your eyes and take several deep breaths while your hand is over your heart or your abdomen. Let your shoulders drop and unclench your jaw. Tell yourself that you are safe, you are strong, and you are worthy of being healed. Imagine standing at the beginning of a beautiful path. The temperature is perfect, and the surroundings are a peaceful reminder of calm. Once you feel safe and supported, tap into that feeling to mark the start of your future.

Step 3: With your eyes still closed, picture the future you want. Ask yourself what healing looks like. What kind of peace do you want to feel? What do you want to create in the future? You may be visualizing holding a baby, snuggling a new puppy, laughing freely with friends and family, or working at a new job. Maybe none of those things appear, and instead you are sitting on a comfortable couch next to someone you love. Go with whatever shows up.

Step 4: Feel the emotions that come over you. Whatever they may be, allow time for your brain and body to remember that you can feel again. Now imagine that you could travel in time, and it is one or two years later. Your future self is walking toward the present day you. The future you has already survived the stages of grief and everything else that comes with it. Future you smiles, but what else is apparent? Are they holding something, and do they want you to know something? Maybe they whisper to you like you haven't lost everything, or there is more joy on the way, this feeling doesn't last forever, or you are stronger than you think. Let those words sink in, take a few deep breaths, and open your eyes.

Step 5: Capture the moment. You can do this by writing a note to yourself, drawing what you saw, or even making a playlist of songs that capture the spirit of the experience. Although you may carry loss, you can also carry hope. Adopting a positive mindset can work wonders when it comes to creating visualizations for the future.

UNRESOLVED GRIEF: WHEN PAIN RESURFACES

Grief has a peculiar tendency to echo through time. Long after closure seems attainable, it can resurface, slipping into your emotional being without notice and leaving lingering shadows upon your heart. Anniversaries, specific milestones, or even seemingly trivial happenings can reawaken dormant feelings with stubborn intensity, reminding you again of an enduring love.

Confronting unresolved grief calls for revealing past healing efforts alongside present emotional needs. Therapy remains an invaluable resource, offering a protected space to process deep-seated grief through guided support. Therapists help traverse convoluted emotions while providing bespoke strategies that resonate with personal experiences. Additionally, community support groups offer consolation through connection. Connecting with others who have experienced similar situations promotes the realization that life is far from solitary.

Signals of unresolved grief indicate the necessity for rudimentary intervention. Avoidance, whether it be evasive of specific reminders or hesitant towards topics related to your loss, frequently indicates unprocessed emotions yearning for attention. Continued sorrow suggests underlying aspects demanding a deeper focus.

Accepting professional support means that certain wounds need care beyond personal capability. Tackling unsettled grief with openness and compassion is needed. Grief-oriented therapy alleviates complexities, extending restorative support for further healing. It can help to ensure the magnification of emotional maturity.

Next up, we will dive into strategies for confronting everyday triggers stemming from social exchanges or introspections, empowering you to see that you can make an emotional comeback through each step on your way to heal a broken heart.

MANAGING TRIGGERS: COPING WITH SOCIAL SITUATIONS

After experiencing a miscarriage or analogous loss, reentering social interactions can seem daunting and full of potential triggers. Events like baby showers or even casual discussions surrounding pregnancy can evoke a cascade of emotions, reopening feelings once thought assuaged. These encounters can render public interactions harrowing, expanding emotional sensitivities into seemingly mundane conversations.

Managing such triggers effectively requires foresight and preparation. Preparing responses for inevitable questions about familial aspirations allows you to guide conversations towards safer topics. Crafting general responses safeguards emotional well-being and preserves the integrity of relationships. Communicating boundaries, whether it involves declining invitations to specific events or excusing yourself early, shows self-respect and emotional security. Friends who are gracious will accommodate these needs.

Want a more specific example of preparation? If you plan to attend an outing, set an alarm on your phone to ensure you make an early exit. You can set the alarm for 45 minutes to an hour after your arrival. As soon as the alarm goes off, leave! You have other obligations that require your attention, so make your exit quickly and quietly if it suits you. Assess the emotional energy dedicated to these engagements, balancing external participation against internal serenity. This form of preparation is needed to keep your mental health moving in a positive direction. After you do this, pat yourself on the back for enduring a social outing. It's all about small wins.

In handling emotionally charged social encounters, prioritizing self-care is a requirement. Offer yourself brief respites when emotions skyrocket. Allow it to be a stolen moment of silence or a breath of fresh air to help you regain composure. Prioritizing individual well-being over conforming to social expectations can become a cornerstone of mental health maintenance. The importance of putting self-care ahead of all things while in social settings cannot be emphasized enough.

Enlist a supportive ally to assist you with social interactions. Their companionship provides reassurance, whether helping to deflect challenging conversations or simply offering a steady presence. Select friends or family members who listen nonjudgmentally and respect your need to withdraw if necessary.

Prepare for potential social challenges. Create rituals that sustain emotional balance. Grab something tangible like a trinket or a cute bracelet to ground yourself during times when emotions are rugged. This will act as a reminder of your inner strength.

Everyday triggers can be a challenge to overcome when they present themselves, but there are methods to disengage from negative feelings. Not all triggers will present themselves in social settings. They may wait to appear while you are in the privacy of your own home. For instance, you may find an article of clothing that was worn the day of the miscarriage or during a happier time of the pregnancy. Just seeing the clothing could release a flood of emotions unexpectedly and drastically turn your mood sour. It may be a good idea to pack away such distinct pieces so they are not easily visible in your closet. You can always return to using them later.

Distraction can be a powerful tool to keep your mind busy in times when silence is deafening. Triggers can be all around you, so having something to keep you occupied helps move you out of a state of guilt and sorrow and into one where you have a task at hand to complete. You may see a pregnant woman while flipping through channels on the TV to find something to watch. If you see this and it is triggering, try looking around the room you are in and find 10 things that have a square shape. For additional distractions, look for 10 other things that are either a particular color or 10 things that start with the same letter.

Over time, distinct personalized strategies will emerge, offering navigation guides for social domains, capturing triumphs alongside setbacks. Celebrate incremental victories, each a testament to enduring strength. Support from loved ones can enable social encounters filled with compassion and determination, reinforcing the ability to bounce back and equipping you with the strength to confront challenges unabatedly.

COMMUNICATING WITH FAMILY AND FRIENDS: SETTING BOUNDARIES

In the immediate aftermath of miscarriage, communicating with well-intentioned family and friends can be both challenging and necessary. While their intentions are often to provide comfort, unsolicited advice or opinions can inadvertently amplify emotional distress. It is key during this period to establish boundaries that safeguard your mental and emotional wellness while preserving the integrity of these relationships.

Boundaries are not about isolating yourself from others but rather about creating safe and supportive environments where your emotions are respected and honored. By setting clear boundaries, you can manage interactions so they support rather than hinder your process of healing. This empowers situational control, enabling you to engage with lenity while prioritizing self-care.

Consider setting boundaries around topics that trigger discomfort or pain. Clearly delineating subjects you prefer not to discuss, such as future pregnancy plans or intricate details of your loss, serves both as self-preservation and an assertion of personal agency. Declining invitations to gatherings like baby showers may be necessary when confronting spaces that could magnify your grief. These personal decisions transform participation from social obligation to choices of personal protection.

Articulate boundaries with clarity and respect. Employ direct yet compassionate language when communicating with others. For example, "I appreciate your concern, but this topic is difficult for me at the moment," conveys your needs without alienating those who wish to help. Such discussions promote awareness about your emotional boundaries while asserting your right to exercise emotional agency.

You may encounter resistance or objection in your boundary setting efforts. Some family or friends might interpret boundaries as a form of distancing, responding with guilt inducing comments aimed at preserving familiar interactions. It is imperative to remain resolute in the face of such responses. Balance care with assertiveness by acknowledging their viewpoint while reaffirming your boundary. Responses such as, "I know you mean well, but this is important for my emotional well-being right now," validate their intentions without relinquishing your agency.

Boundaries should be versatile and evolve along your road to wellness. Regular assessment ensures they remain appropriate and strengthens your commitment to emotional health. This flexibility enables you to modify interactions constructively, rooted in continuous reinforcement of your emotional wellness.

When boundaries are respected, interactions become grounded in interchangeable care rather than stress, reshaping relationships into genuine support conduits. Open, respectful communication regarding these boundaries transforms interactions, resulting in environments where confusion is minimized and support and trust flourish.

Setting boundaries equates to an act of self-love, asserting your worth during times of emotional revolt. It draws a clear marker during unsettling times, prioritizing your peace alongside the needs of others with grace and wisdom. Embrace the courage in setting these boundaries, affirming that vulnerability necessitates protection, and boundaries act as expressions of respect and empowerment.

Actionable Item: Boundary Setting Exercise

Reflect on prior situations where you felt uncomfortable or overwhelmed due to someone's words or actions surrounding your loss. Use this reflection to practice setting boundaries:

- Situation:

  _____

- Boundary statement:

  _____

Rehearse articulating this boundary confidently, preparing you to express your needs effectively and with grace when needed. Such foresight and practice empower you to uphold emotional boundaries with ease and conviction. Remember, establishing healthy boundaries requires an ongoing commitment from all involved, as well as openness to re-evaluation over time. You will find that not everyone may instantly comprehend or support your needs. Patience and persistence are necessary for transition and adaptation.

HANDLING INSENSITIVE COMMENTS: BUILDING RESILIENCE

After experiencing a miscarriage, one might face well-meaning comments that inadvertently hurt. Despite the intentions, expressions like "everything happens for a reason" or "you can try again" might seem dismissive. Such remarks can leave you feeling misunderstood and isolated. Anticipating these moments by recognizing potential triggers can prepare you emotionally, empowering you to turn hurtful interactions into opportunities for self-advocacy and boundary setting.

Responding graciously to insensitive comments can be empowering. Consider calm, factual replies that reflect your feelings without escalating tension. Saying something like, "I appreciate your concern, but I find it difficult to discuss this topic," sets boundaries while remaining courteous. Sometimes, self-care might mean choosing to leave the conversation to protect your emotional well-being. This step is operational self-care, not retreat. Prioritizing mental health by distancing yourself from distressing encounters is both legitimate and necessary.

These comments likely evoke an emotional response, possibly igniting grief or anger, destabilizing your healing course. Mindfulness, as previously introduced, can aid in processing these emotions constructively. Taking a deep breath before replying or finding a quiet corner to gather your thoughts allows you time to regain composure. Mindfulness encourages awareness of the present, creating space between stimulus and reaction. This practice yields the buildup of your power, fortifying your capacity to manage challenging conversations with poise.

Surrounding yourself with caring individuals is instrumental in building resistance to insensitive remarks. A circle of empathetic friends and family offers a safehouse where you can express feelings sans retribution. These confidants refrain from providing unsolicited advice and offer the support and space you need to grieve in comfort. Constructing such a network ensures that healing isn't a desolate thing, but something buoyed by those who uplift your vitality.

ENHANCING COMMUNICATION SKILLS

Communication after a miscarriage can be fragile and emotionally charged. Challenges can present themselves when communicating with a partner, friends, medical professionals, and even random strangers in public. Reclaim and enhance your voice after loss by starting with self-compassionate speech. If you are blaming yourself or silencing your pain at the behest of others, try replacing that internal monologue with gentle self-talk. Instead of telling yourself that you should be over this by now, be reminded that grief does not have a timeline. Instead of feeling like you don't want to bother anyone, remind yourself that you too deserve support and connection.

Get comfortable with the idea that you can name your needs without having any guilt attached to them. Unapologetically express those needs clearly to get your point across. For example, "I appreciate your support, but I am not ready to talk about my loss" or "I feel _ when _ happens. What I need right now is _."

The response that you receive from others may range from acceptance to confusion and everything in between. Whatever the response, know that it is not a reflection of your worth or the validity of your grief. Having a safe circle of people who know, listen, respect your boundaries, and make you feel more like your regular self is important. Even if your circle is down to one person, that one person could make a huge difference in your emotional well-being.

Strengthening your communication repertoire involves proactive skills. Enrolling in workshops or webinars that emphasize conflict resolution or empathetic communication builds confidence. These sessions can offer role playing scenarios to practice and refine your response strategies. Obtaining these skills enables you to approach challenging conversations with clarity and control, enhancing emotional and social competence in testing situations.

Actionable Item: Crafting Your Response Toolkit

Consider developing a personal toolkit for handling insensitive comments. Reflect on past exchanges and identify strategies that have worked well. Note these responses in a journal or save them on your phone for easy reference. This tactic empowers you with pre-considered replies, metamorphosing vulnerability into expressions of empowerment and self-assurance.

CHAPTER 3
PHYSICAL RECOVERY: CARING FOR YOUR BODY AFTER LOSS

UNDERSTANDING POSTPARTUM PHYSICAL SYMPTOMS

EVERY MISCARRIAGE IS as unique as the individuals experiencing it. The body embarks on a universal course of healing and restoration with each symptom representative of a marker on this route. Miscarriage can feel disorienting, a loss compounded by physical reminders of what was and the bittersweet return to a pre-pregnant state. Being cognizant of these symptoms bestows a semblance of control and empowerment in the thick of grief.

The onset of vaginal bleeding, often a precursor of this unchosen transition, marks the body's course to natural realignment. Light spotting may gradually escalate into a heavier flow. The duration and intensity remain unpredictable, sometimes spanning anywhere from a few days to several weeks. Accompanying bleeding and abdominal cramping signals the body's proactive expulsion of pregnancy tissues. These contractions, albeit painful, mirror your reproductive system's restorative dance back to equilibrium.

Equally important is being cognizant of symptoms that warrant immediate medical intervention. Not all postpartum experiences follow the textbook way. Heavy bleeding, defined as more than one soaked pad per hour, alongside severe, unmanageable pain, acts as an alarm highlighting the potential need for medical support. Such symptoms could indicate complications such as retained tissue or infection, requiring timely medical attention to safeguard your well-being and ease the restoration process.

Fatigue, both physical and emotional, weaves into the post-partum forum. While the body demands rest and patience, hidden layers of emotional loss manifest through physical fatigue, reinforcing the necessity for the gentleness of personal custody. Acknowledging the link between your physical recovery and mental state, and approaching it with compassion, sets the foundation for a healing journey charac-terized by empathy.

The emotional reverberations of physical symptoms further complicate this grand recovery. Each cramp, each drop of blood, can trigger emotional echoes of sadness, which may translate to you as vivid echoes of your prior hopes and dreams. Confirming this associated string of events validates the integrity of your grief, allowing the emotions to parlay into healing avenues. In these moments, holistically addressing your physical and emotional scopes can soothe you, creating ways to mend and embrace the intricacies of dealing with loss.

Attuning to your body's needs involves responding to its signals without conjecture. Embrace rest when required and nourish your form and spirit with sincere kindness. Seeking support from loved ones or professionals becomes urgent, divulging the challenging duality of physical healing and emotional grieving. By leaning into your support network and sharing your troubles, you nurture a synergistic yearning for purpose. Mastering the art of knowing when companionship or solitude serves your healing best is a valuable lesson.

Integrating calming activities can be beneficial between the layers of grief and the unpredictable nature of physical recuperation. Engage with creative outlets such as adult coloring books, drawing, or other artistic expressions. Allow these to become constructive channels for emotions, providing balance and renewed purpose. Incorporating these outlets within your support plan engrains protectiveness against chaos, offering shelter and purpose during days otherwise defined by uncertainty.

Healing reveals itself as a byway of varied pieces, moving away from straight, predictable timelines towards a track that honors the unique pace and needs of each individual. Every step forward embodies heart, rebirthing your link to a physical existence intersecting with lived experience. Throughout this landscape, extend compassion to yourself, savoring restful, introspective periods as inherent parts of this trail. Embrace this union as a record of reconstruction, where body and spirit integrate, fortifying one another in heartfelt cycles of renewal.

Though daunting, recovery after a miscarriage is simultaneously ripe with prospects for rejuvenation and personal evolution. Armed with understanding and compassion, you can draw upon the well of inner strength, propelling yourself toward wholeness with the grace and courage necessary to walk through loss into renewal.

EMOTIONAL HEALING THROUGH PHYSICAL ACTIVITY

Engaging in a physical activity such as booking and attending a session in a smash room provides a therapeutic avenue for healing emotional wounds. Smash rooms (also known as rage rooms) are safety focused environments designed to allow participants to gear up in personal protective equipment like a hard hat with mask, gloves, and coveralls, and then use tools like hammers and baseball bats to smash glass and electronics. This type of specialized controlled chaos encourages external expression of internal unrest, translating elaborate feelings into tangible forms. Some participants attend these venting sessions alone, while others opt to have a partner or small group join them.

Smash rooms are gaining in popularity around the world. There are hundreds of them in the United States alone. Physical exertion in a smash room can lower stress levels and simultaneously provide entertainment. Endorphins are released, and this promotes improvement in overall well-being. This creative endeavor serves as an emotional proxy, revealing routes to healing that transcend verbal articulation. It offers a respite, a momentary escape into an alternate realm where emotional release is not only possible but encouraged.

NUTRITION FOR RECOVERY: HEALING THROUGH DIET

In nourishing your postpartum body, the significance of diet cannot be overstated. It stands not just as a tool for refueling but as an emblem of governance and revitalization for bodily grief. Engaging in conscious dietary practices carries your body through the continuum of physical and emotional strain inherent within this period.

Replenishing iron levels, disrupted by blood loss, sits at the forefront of nutritional recovery. Lean meats, such as chicken and beef, and plant-based iron sources such as lentils, spinach, and legumes create a rich dietary landscape in this essential mineral. Ingesting iron complements the tangible approach back to strength, building up reserves for tomorrow's toughness. Equally important is the role of vitamin C in supporting tissue repair, enhancing your body's natural healing process. Oranges, grapefruits, strawberries, and vibrant bell peppers, each rich in this vitamin, act as allies, bolstering your healing capacities when woven into your nutrient plan. A colorful, varietal diet, rich in vitamins and minerals, nourishes the physical body and reinforces emotional health through conscious service and personal kindness.

A comprehensive diet accounts for more than isolated nutrients but envelops a panorama of nourishing elements. Wholesome grains, colorful vegetables, and rich proteins compose a palette from which optimal health thrives. Leafy greens support detoxification while offering the intimacy of care that infuses each recovering fiber with life. Hydration joins this symphony as a cornerstone, with water supporting digestion and maintaining energy reserves, ensuring your body remains attuned to recovery's rhythm.

In scenarios where dietary intake alone may not suffice, dietary supplements may provide invaluable support, always aligned with healthcare guidance. Iron supplements could replenish depleted reserves, while the Omega-3 fatty acids that are often found in fish or flaxseed oils, could alleviate inflammation and render mental clarity. However, discussing new supplements with a trusted healthcare advisor ensures adherence to personalized health plans, aligning holistic guidance with individualized channels.

The emotional magnitude of miscarriage often reverberates into eating patterns, potentially leading to the shadow of emotional eating. While this temporary support may provide a brief distraction, it can also overshadow the abstract healing that comes from mindful nourishment. Embrace mindful eating, the art of attentive engagement, encouraging tacit recognition of hunger cues and the delight of savoring each bite's inherent sustenance. A food journal might reveal new contours in eating habits, casting light on patterns rooted not to hunger but emotional drawbacks. Documenting these revelations enacts a rediscovery of conscious choice in food selection and consumption.

Balancing a diet following loss extends beyond mere consumption. It also embodies satiating through mindful inclusion. By paying attention intently to your body's signals, you establish a relationship with food that cherishes its role in nourishing, one that embraces your inherent toughness and capacity for transformation. New growth is celebrated in the kitchen, each meal a testament to your courageous return to nourishment and life's continuity.

Explore community supported agriculture or local farmer's markets, which create unique bonds through united commitments to holistic well-being. These businesses provide the community with a seamless extension of provisions beyond the kitchen walls to facilitate emotional camaraderie and an earnest sense of belonging within your healing trajectory. The transformative prospects of nutrition are boundless, each meal a moment of intimate reconnection with oneself, designed to provide copious solutions and comfort during raw, evolving times.

GENTLE EXERCISE: RECONNECTING WITH YOUR BODY

Physical movement in terms of postpartum healing serves as both reconciliation with your body and a step towards reclaiming your physical autonomy. Gentle exercise blends seamlessly as part of physical rehabilitation and emotional equilibrium restoration. By introducing exercise, you invite the release of endorphins, nature's inherent mood enhancers, bestowing glimpses of lightness in grief. Movement acts as a counter to lethargy, spliced with emotional weight. Regular exercise reinvigorates, feeding both body and spirit. Through this incorporation, you claim a fortified influence over your body's newfound healing.

Exercise selection during this sensitive juncture underscores consideration, as sensitivity reigns supreme. Walking, particularly within the symphony of nature, offers spirited renewal and peace. The rhythmic cadence experienced through each step, coupled with natural tranquility, gives rise to reflective exploration. Alternatively, light yoga or stretching exercises create gentle avenues for relieving tension and achieving flexibility. Through these practices, mindfulness arises, keeping you in present bodily awareness without overwhelming exertion. For many, these exercise modalities encapsulate physical nurture while harmonizing emotional ease, creating symbiotic, holistic recovery opportunities.

Listen to your body's messages as you start exercising after a miscarriage. Each person's healing approach is as diverse as the range of comfort and discomfort they encounter. The practice of tuning in to discomfort, paired with respectful adjustments to intensity, solidifies a trustful, caring relationship towards your own body. Listening becomes fertile ground where healing, connection, and renewed staunchness take root, particularly following loss.

Motivation can waver in exercise endeavors, particularly during emotional flux. Build small, attainable goals to provide structure and motivation. Start with brief walks or concise yoga sessions, gradually increasing the length of time as comfort evolves. Every minor triumph stands as a testament to your persistence and determination. Enlisting a workout companion enhances motivation through companionship and accountability. Sharing these endeavors with someone who comprehends the depth of your pain layers additional encouragement, rendering the drive forward seemingly less insurmountable.

During intervals when motivation wanes, remind yourself of exercise's boundless benefits in caring for the mind, body, and soul. Maintaining a progress journal serves as a reflective tool, allowing you to observe your emotional landscape before and after exercise sessions. By unveiling the gradual, meaningful transformations within, your diary affirms each small victory within your larger recovery landscape.

Connecting with group classes or online communities can harness support. These platforms offer structured, programmatic approaches suited to your needs while playing into companionship. Here, a give and take exchange of reflections, movement, and discussions creates a collaborative unit of healing, infusing fortitude across symbiotic, personal spaces.

Exercise fuels physical flexibility and acts as a channel to reestablish self after the deeply felt loss. Each physical session embodies inner strength and commitment, nursing your body and spirit across emotional landscapes. As you integrate exercise more deeply into your daily routine, allow movement to represent your journey, recognizing your inner strength as a shining example of how shattered aspirations can evolve from loss to resilience in the face of adversity. Integrating gentle exercise into your daily routine post-miscarriage might initially serve as an intentional act, but may evolve organically into foundational aspects of healing. These practices can offer peace during times of uncertainty and aspiration during moments of sorrow. Entrust the rhythm of movement to guide you like a beacon illuminating the gateway to internal reconnection.

HOLISTIC HEALTH APPROACHES: INTEGRATING ALTERNATIVE THERAPIES

Embarking on holistic health paths in the aftermath of a miscarriage could provide soothing complements to conventional medical care, harmonizing the healing spectrum. Holistic methodologies envelop the individual as a composite of body, mind, and spirit, emphasizing the robust echoes within these elements. Acupuncture, steeped in ancient wisdom, is one method utilized for alleviating stress and facilitating tranquility. Targeted stimulation of key bodily points achieves tension relief, and an opportunity for the restoration of balance emerges. This calming approach presents a velvety portal to address both physical ailments and emotional imbroglios. Though debated in efficacy, acupuncture has been considered by some as a complementary approach to improve hormonal balance and fertility following a miscarriage.

Massage therapy provides another avenue for recovery, focusing on stress reduction through physically therapeutic engagement. As muscle tension dissolves under gentle pressure, circulation flourishes, allowing the spirit to align towards wellness. Enhanced by tranquil settings, massage therapy serves as a haven for reconnection and peaceful relief. Herbal remedies, such as chamomile and lavender, are infused with gentle, sedative qualities that nudge anxiety aside and encourage restful slumber. Delicate chamomile tea before bedtime might serve as an emissary of tranquility. Exploring supplementary treatments and supportive therapies enriches the available management spectrum. Aromatherapy, too, is embraced by some for its potential to alleviate emotional distress through soothing scents, encouraging relaxation and tranquility.

Emerging therapies, filled with potential, call for a lively discussion with healthcare providers prior to incorporating them into your recovery process. Even discussions regarding herbal remedies safeguard against potential medication interactions or conditions. Professional insights render tailored therapeutic experiences, embodying traditional and complementary techniques under one harmonious umbrella. Integrating holistic therapies harmonizes with conventional medical advice, offering foundations for inclusive healing. This convergence taps into a spectrum awareness of recovery, embracing body and spirit's reciprocities alongside traditional support.

Guide yourself using personal intuition. Follow your body's harmonious wisdom, encourage curiosity, and welcome exploration through these therapeutic lanes. Selections align with self-knowledge, honoring the recovery period's transitions as they embody both physical and emotional healing into symphonic movement.

Holistic health interventions deliver the nexus of ancient and modern insight, engendering empowerment throughout healing processes. Integration creates sanctuaries for body and mind during recovery, gaining staying power as testament to the capacity for renewal within a saddening loss. Holistic travels affirm unique healing voyages and are catalysts for transformation and courageous emergent growth. Embrace these stages, patient in their gifts and organic in their evolution. Holistic methodologies highlight the communal aspect of healing by bridging personal insights with the broader idea of pooled well-being.

HANDLING MEDICAL FOLLOW-UPS: WHAT TO EXPECT

Within postpartum recovery, medical follow-ups surface as foundational checkpoints along your healing expedition. Despite the anxiety that coincides with these appointments, recognizing their significance reframes them from nominal duties to integral components of body management.

Be mindful that the environment of an OBGYN office can cause emotional triggers to swell expeditiously. While in the waiting area, you are likely to see patients in varying stages of pregnancy, and that can be difficult to digest, especially if your loss was very recent. If you find it too difficult to remain seated in the waiting area, let the check-in staff know that you need to step out and have them call you on your cell phone once you are ready to be seen. Be sure to stay in the immediate area, like the parking lot or an exterior hallway, so that you can quickly return to the office upon your name being called. Compassionate staff will gladly accommodate your request. In the event you feel emotionally stable enough to remain in the general waiting area, use a distraction to keep your mind from racing. You could scroll through social media, browse websites for random online window shopping for something unrelated to the situation such as fancy glass-ware sets or garden tools, or even text someone in your support circle.

A significant function of follow-up lies in ensuring complete uterine recovery, underscoring the natural transition by confirming complete expulsion of pregnancy tissue. These appointments also graciously address emotional hurdles, aligning physical with mental processes. Providers can suggest resources or referrals to help you beyond the clinical sphere, promoting comprehensive restoration.

Follow-up visits typically incorporate several assessments ensuring your holistic health. Ultrasound examinations, noninvasive by nature, confirm full miscarriage recovery, uncovering potential complications due to retained tissue. Routine blood tests accompany even more integral checks, monitoring hormone declines. Specifically, hCG levels diminish, demonstrating hormonal reversion pre-pregnancy. This is an observable hallmark of your physiological restoration.

Preparation facilitates empowerment during consultations, sustaining collaboration between patient and provider. Pose informed inquiries regarding future pregnancy, if anticipated. Gaining a clear understanding of the risks, precautions, and plans for the future can provide thoughtful insight. Discuss any ongoing symptoms, bridging communication to approach coexisting physical and emotional states confidently.

Harness recovery tracking through health journals, which add context to your follow ups. Document physical symptoms and emotional reflections to gauge where you are. Appointments evolve into multidimensional assessments, collecting data on both physical and mental well-being. Feel empowered by active engagement, ensuring that each visit encompasses your needs. Authentic exchanges demonstrate personalized components, sparking confidence and calm.

Approach these visits as partnerships with healthcare providers, enhancing recovery customs through joint engagement. Appointments become reflective spaces, creating leeway to comprehensive support sources. Exploring continuation of support groups or mental health counseling exemplifies holistic healing as a pursuit to honor the unique dimensions of individual revival. Actively engage, enforcing a routine revisitation notion embedding mind-body care integration. This partnership defines the shape for your holistic recovery orbit, uniting complementary resources into cohesive support.

ADDRESSING PHYSICAL AND EMOTIONAL INTERCONNECTION

Grief is decipherable as a complicated blend of physical sensations and emotional experiences, intertwining in a deeply kindred way. Attending to this synergy is central in recovering from miscarriage, acknowledging that interconnected strategies thread through holistic revival.

Physical symptoms like cramping and fatigue trigger emotional responses, unblurring the boundary between body and mind. Emotions such as sadness, frustration, or guilt magnify awareness of physical presence, affixing each twinge as phenomenal reflections of deeper yearning. Recognizing this mind-body union directs empathetic recovery efforts toward multidimensional planes.

Exercise, an indomitable ally against physical tension and mental fatigue, lifts spirits through endorphin infusion. Accumulated achievements generate renewed control and assurance through small steps. Short workouts are great mood boosters. Holistic recovery advances through body wide experiences, both emotional and physical. Daily mindfulness backs perspectives, grounding mental commotion across stormy skies through observational patience. Present focused engagement calms alternating tempests, offering gentle glimmers of clarity among restlessness. Integrating holistic support by embodying dual needs embeds common ground therapeutic avenues, underpinning modalities fostering emotional equilibrium at every stage. Complementing mind and body dimensions, acupuncture and yoga act in concert with cosmic complements during the healing symphony. Shaping holistic periods, practicing mind-body synchronization, and aligning remedies as trusted supports.

Dialogue enriches engagement with healthcare providers, avowing emotional dimensions after a miscarriage. Presenting emotional chronicles in clinical discussions ensures personalized, courageously sculpted care strategies. Open discourse inspires adaptive approaches, converging on healing strategies driven by compassionate partnership.

Maintaining this delicate balance requires keen awareness of the allied stories of mind and body, promoting a well-informed journey of healing that fully embraces a holistic approach to wellness. Honoring an appreciation of this healing process allows for a more natural and gradual untangling of both physical and emotional hardships. The fused relationship between mind and body establishes a solid foundation for healing. Focusing on this connection enhances the continuity of healing, creating broader, personalized avenues for getting through grief.

Actionable Item: Physical and Emotional Support Plan

Crafting an individualized support plan becomes a sound strategy in provisioning both your physical and emotional landscapes. Engage in keeping a reflective journal. Document symptoms and correlate them to your evolving emotional states. As you track bleeding or cramping, also record how they sway your mental outlook from day to day. This exercise not only assists in monitoring physical recovery but highlights emotional fluctuations, patterns that could emerge through your notes.

CHAPTER 4
BUILDING SUPPORT SYSTEMS: FINDING AND OFFERING HELP

REACHING OUT: HOW TO ASK FOR AND RECEIVE HELP

VERBALIZING the need for help is a big step. It is of utmost importance to recognize when you need additional support. Doing your part to eliminate the stigma behind asking for assistance may be a big ask, but you can do it. Initially, you may be reluctant, but that's okay. Even those of us who are looked upon as a pillar of support for our friends and family need guidance too. Common signs to look for to determine if you or someone you know needs help include trouble completing simple tasks, frequent bouts of forgetfulness, and constant irritability.

Effective communication can make the task of asking for help more palatable. A technique for clearly articulating needs and feelings to potential supporters includes the use of "I" statements to express needs. For example, "I need help making dinner", or "I would like you to pick my child up from school" directly convey needs. Be sure to practice active listening to facilitate reciprocated clarity.

OVERCOMING BARRIERS TO ASKING FOR HELP

Some of us experience emotional and psychological barriers that may prevent us from seeking help. It could be cloaked as the fear of burdening others, or even as a fear of appearing vulnerable. The use of effective communication as described above can assist individuals in circumventing these road-blocks. As time progresses, it will become easier to get past these hurdles. Furthermore, learning to accept help and keeping your ears open to guidance from others will serve you well in the long run.

Several other factors could influence whether someone has a barrier to asking for help. It all comes down to fear. The fear of rejection is real, even from those who personally know you well. The fear of nominal energy drain keeps one from reaching out, as does the fear of change or losing control of a situation. Fear also has physical effects on the body. Blood flow shifts towards muscles in preparation for a fight or flight response, your heart rate increases, and trembling or nausea may occur. The combination of these effects could be a seemingly impossible hurdle in asking for help.

BUILDING YOUR SUPPORT NETWORK: WHO TO TURN TO

In times of devastating grief and loss, the emotional tides can feel relentless and overwhelming. It is during these moments that the human need for connection becomes most apparent. Recognizing and growing a network of support can transform these raging times into an experience marked by collective strength and enduring compassion. The individuals who form your support network might be diverse. Each could offer unique help, from emotional consolation to practical assistance.

Identifying the right allies begins with observing and ascertaining who genuinely can participate in your life without being discerning. Genuine altruism from a confidant allows you to process your feelings without fear of being misread. Consider friends who have consistently demonstrated an open-hearted presence. Their ability to sit with you in moments of silence or engage in deep, meaningful conversations is priceless. They offer the precious gift of presence, a steady rock through the commotion to bring you into a renewed version of yourself.

Consciously affirming the roles these individuals play in your life can be a grounding practice. No person can be everything to everyone, but recognizing the specific qualities and strengths that each member of your support network brings not only aids your personal healing but also empowers your supporters. These positions, whether it is your friend's knack for making you laugh or your mother's ability to offer a different perspective that you never considered, are crucial in shaping a support network that feels both personalized and deeply interconnected. With every bit of gratitude shown for these acts, these relationships are either furthered or initiated, deepening alliances through appreciation and common respect.

A sound support system's hallmark is founded on empathy and built with patience, trust, and active listening standards. Those who stand with you in sorrow often possess the rare ability to hear beyond spoken words, perceiving the emotions tangled beneath them. This makes way for the elements of trust and openness, meaningful ingredients for healing. The steady calm they bring becomes particularly vital during times when grief is expressed in unpredictable ways, reminding you that it's okay for healing to have an indiscriminate style, with steps taken back and forth in the dance of recovery.

Effective communication becomes the lifeline that underwrites these relationships. When you're able to articulate your needs, such as a desire for company or a request for solitude, you pave the way for comprehension. Communicating openly about these needs gleans a joint respect where neither party feels lost or unwanted. For example, simple statements like "I need a salad for lunch today" or "Could you join me for a walk?" establish clear expectations and prevent misinterpretations. Open dialogues invite collaborative backing, ensuring your emotional landscape is declared and respected.

Investment in these relationships is equally important and involves continuous reciprocity. Announce the contributions of your support circle. Uphold gratitude by expressing appreciation for their presence and actions, like sending a heartfelt message or spending time together. Engaging in routines that reinforce these bonds, be it cooking together or participating in group hobbies, builds intrepidity within the relationship. These activities secure your connection in positive experiences, serving as reminders of the joy and comfort that can exist alongside healing.

Furthermore, consider what unique qualities each person brings to your support system. Whether lending an ear or providing hands on help, becoming aware of these dynamics strengthens your ability to lean on them effectively and reinforce those unions. Recognizing and harnessing the synergy of diverse strengths transforms your support network into a powerful force of collaboration and love.

Your connection with them, however, should be reciprocal. While leaning on them in moments of need, offering your presence and support during their challenges deepens these relationships. This complementary exchange holds dear a culture of compassion, building a network of connections that strengthens each participant. As you check in on them and recognize their efforts, you create a supportive environment that champions relationship growth. Feel the strength of the kinship during these interactions. They represent an invisible safety net designed to catch and lift you again. By advancing these relationships, you champion a culture of correlative presence and stamina, creating a circle of support that sustains healing through its spirited blend of grace and kind-heartedness.

An open embrace of mutual emotions binds you together, affirming that these relationships offer both healing and the prospect of something great on the horizon. Friends and family become beams of light against the shadows, promoting the methodology toward healing filled with companionship and good nature. Through thoughtful reflection, open communication, and matching care, you chart a course toward creating a strong support system. This is a testament to the idea that even in the darkest times, together, we are not alone.

EFFECTIVE WAYS TO OFFER GENUINE SUPPORT

The impact of genuine support from family and friends shall not go unnoticed. A sibling might intuitively step into the role of caretaker, handling daily responsibilities to ease your load. Meanwhile, a parent could offer the familiar comfort of home cooked meals, each bite grounding you in the warmth of remembered love. A neighbor could take your dog for a walk once daily for a week to give you more time to relax. These people have shared history and can provide comforting familiarity that is needed during your hardships. The roles they play blend practicality with emotional support, recognizing the duality of healing as both nurturing and liberating.

A substantial component of communication within any support network is the ability to listen actively. Listening goes beyond hearing words. It involves comprehending not only what is being said, but also the context and underlying emotions. A good listener creates a safe space where the speaker feels valued and understood. In active listening, attention is keenly focused on the speaker, with interruptions kept at bay, questions posed thoughtfully, and feedback given constructively. Through such interactions, support networks transform from passive circles of association into hearty ecosystems of healing and empowerment.

Partners play a decisive role in support as well, and there are additional ways genuine support can be offered. With your permission and when you feel ready, your partner could take the lead in researching and contacting therapists for your individual sessions. From experience, I can say that this is ultimately how I ended up in therapy. I have a common insurance plan, but finding a qualified therapist in my area who (1) accepted my insurance and (2) had available appointments in a reasonable time versus a six-month waitlist was challenging. On two separate occasions during Year 1 and Year 2 of my three-year grieving period, I spent almost an hour making phone calls and leaving voicemails for therapists in the pursuit of grief counseling. Those unsuccessful attempts were nearly enough to drive me over the edge and always ended in tears. Some of the tears were even left on voicemails. I cried every single day during the first year. My husband had been encouraging me to seek out counseling opportunities from the very beginning, but I was largely not committed to accepting that level of help. During Year 3, he encouraged me to seek professional counseling again, and he even printed out a list of locations nearby. Calls were made to a few but again, the waitlist issue kept coming up. My husband recommended that I try using the Employee Assistance Program (EAP) from my job, as most employers offer free anonymous programs and services for mental health counseling. I took his advice, which led me to the start of my first therapy sessions. I will be forever grateful for my husband's continued push towards therapy, as well as the two therapists who helped me climb out of depression.

Your support network can show up for you in ways that may seem small to them, yet they perform acts of service that restore your spirit. Below are more ways to support someone going through a miscarriage:

- Start a meal train for them so fresh, cooked food is delivered to their home for three weeks or so.
- Transport their children to and from school activities for a few weeks.
- Drop off grocery essentials at their front door once a week for a month. Include items like paper towels, facial tissue, a bag of fresh fruit, and a guilty pleasure like a candy bar.

- Accompany them to medical follow-up appointments. These are in high stress environments and just sitting in the waiting area can trigger unsavory emotions.
- Gift comforts like new fuzzy slippers or a soft, fleece blanket
- Acknowledge that miscarriage is emotional and mood swings may be frequent. Be prepared to take that into consideration and refrain from taking anything personal.
- Obtain a supply of sanitary pads and over the counter painkillers to help with the physical side effects of miscarriage.
- Provide a quiet activity to work on such as a book of crossword puzzles or an adult coloring book with colored pencils. This can be used during times of insomnia.
- Ask them what they would like you to do specifically. Avoid using the phrase, "Let me know if I can do anything for you," as that tends to result in inaction.

Actionable Item: Identifying Your Support Network

Take a moment to gaze inward and consider who surrounds you with genuine reasoning and kindness:

- Who among your friends consistently offers empathetic, nonjudgmental listening?
- Which family members have respected your boundaries while providing major support?
- Who exhibits patience and genuine kindness, especially during your most challenging times?

Write their names down, recognize the roles they play in your life, and reflect on how you can maintain open channels of communication with them. These reflections help you clearly identify the champions of support in your life, giving you a clearer sense of who you can rely on.

PARTNER PERSPECTIVES: THE SILENT GRIEVERS

Miscarriage affects more than the pregnant woman. Partners traverse their unique meetings with grief often quietly. The challenge lies in balancing their own emotional uprising with the required support role. Many feel an overwhelming helplessness; their ability to change the past or ease their partner's suffering is nullified. This helplessness can shift into exclusionary feelings as partners move through a grief landscape, often lacking a roadmap or explicit role.

Societal expectations amplify this struggle, obligating partners, especially men, to stand as unfaltering supporters. Cultural norms traditionally cast partners as the stoic caregiver, prompting them to suppress personal grief to uphold a strong family facade. This mandate can spark an internal clash between the personal desire to mourn and the external pressure to display unswerving strength.

Partner stories inject a voice into the muted struggle within this quiet territory. One partner can derive strength from peer groups, where unified experiences offer clarity and civility. Within these spaces, they lay out coping strategies without conviction, underscoring the critical need for communities that recognize vulnerability and validate partner grief.

Facilitating partners' healing requires them to embark on their own journey. Joining support groups crafted for partners opens a relaxed sanctuary for candid feelings sharing. These groups offer connection threads with those seizing partner specific challenges. They afford partners space to articulate feelings obscured elsewhere. Grief navigation demands patience and compassion for partners. Recognizing the legitimacy of their pain is critical for their healing. Locating expressive and supportive spaces ensures they nourish their grief with dignity, enhancing personal and relational growth.

ENCOURAGING PARTNER INCLUSIVE HEALING SPACES

Establishing partner inclusive healing spaces involves integrating partner specific rituals into gatherings or support systems. It says we are a team, and we are healing together. Promoting open dialogues about their emotions within community events validates their experiences, enhancing their connection to healing efforts. Viewing partners as full participants in the collective grief process affirms both individual and relational recovery, marking a holistic healing approach.

Partners partake in unique exchanges with grief, often overshadowed by societal expectations to maintain strong exteriors. Cultural norms can pressure them to offer support while sidelining their emotions. Sharing their stories shines a light on their struggles and coping methods. Be sure to leave room for both partners' grieving styles to be enacted, and define what healing together looks like in your relationship. Learn things about miscarriage together by watching short videos or listening to a podcast. Normalize what you are going through so that communication can be opened in a nonconfrontational manner. The use of "we" language can also support a partner inclusive healing space. Instead of "I lost the baby," try using "we lost the baby," "we're grieving," or "we're healing together".

UNDERSTANDING PARTNER GRIEF: SUPPORTING EACH OTHER

The heartbreaking experience of miscarriage exerts a profound emotional toll on both partners. Everyone may experience grief in their own way. This shapes their perspectives and coping strategies. It is important to affirm the sophisticated duality of joint and individual grief while learning to commandeer this emotional dimension together as a couple. There may be intervals of role reversal within your relationship, where one partner struggles more than the other, and this can change over time. It is possible to support them through this, even as you are managing personal grief. You can offer to take on additional responsibilities temporarily. Examples of this can include letting your partner know that you will handle all the laundry and food preparation for the rest of the week. You can take things a few days or a week at a time so as not to become overwhelmed.

Each partner carries a unique grief signature. It may be visible in different avenues, with one partner externalizing emotions through tears or conversations, while the other internalizes by withdrawing or appearing stoic. Being aware of these differing expressions is momentous for requited awareness and sensitivity. Recognizing that each response is valid breeds compassion and strengthens your union, honoring the distinct blueprints both of you create.

Open communication is central to sustaining empathy. Engage in meaningful discussion with your partner, planning times to incorporate activities into your lives. This discovery process is about having combined love, compassion, and transformative support while creating a haven to work on your game plan towards healing together. Setting the scene for intentional moments of open dialogue allows partners to express feelings without fear of adjudication or dismissal. In this space, "I feel" statements endow this communication skill by articulating personal emotions, preventing blame or misapprehension. Statements like "I feel now more than ever" promote a culture of vulnerability, inviting both partners to explore needs candidly and collaboratively. Such dialogues create a stronghold where love upholds the core of both individuals.

Sharing these experiences becomes a priority during periods of grief, offering comfort as life presents challenges. A deeper digestion of each other's perspectives is the key to strengthening your partnership, empowering individual and collective recovery. You embrace a technique that cherishes individual and mutual gustiness while celebrating love's enduring strength in grief's shadows through consensual regard and purposeful cultivation of the bond between you.

Beyond conversation, joint healing activities can pull both of you closer together. Attending counseling sessions as a couple opens doors to strength. Under the guidance of a therapist, you encounter an opportunity to explore both individual and common emotions. Here, counselors facilitate communication, offering tailored strategies that uplift your relationship while respecting individual emotions. Joint engagement in mindfulness practices such as walking meditations or breathing exercises together provides additional closeness, linking relaxation with collaborative support.

In addition to therapeutic sessions, consider recreational activities that promote a sense of concord and joy. Whether it's dancing, hiking, or taking a cooking class together, these moments of bonded activity inject vibrancy and distraction, temporarily alleviating the weight of grief. By prioritizing time for playfulness in the shadows of sorrow, both partners gain a reprieve where laughter and levity feature an avenue toward healing.

Notably, partners may navigate their grief at different paces, underscoring the importance of nobility and patience. Providing the space for individual reflection is as important as symbiotic support. There will be moments when one partner needs solitude to process emotions, while another seeks presence. Respect these choices and honor the process by which your partner channels grief. Such patience is a mainstay in your relationship as it signifies honoring the depth of love.

Support is digestible in countless ways, often transcending verbal communication to convey depth and compassion. Small gestures communicate love where language may fall short. This nonverbal communication shows up in the form of a warm embrace, the dual silence of presence, or tackling household tasks together, as symbols of reliability and connection. These acts signal devotion and reinforce a resilient bond where bilateral vigilance enriches both partners in the midst of vulnerability.

Always remember that the loss influences both partners. Participation in this experience deepens your connection, and your cohesiveness conditions concerted healing. By championing each other's needs gracefully, you honor the love underlying grief, reinforcing a bond that flourishes despite uncertainty. Your partnership creates a home for healing, bridging the emotional spectrum with compassion exhibited through actions, words, and loving silence. If both partners are struggling, seek external support to prevent burnout and emotional exhaustion. By recognizing the intense impact miscarriage can have on both partners, you generate a culture of love and compassion throughout this pivotal chapter of life. Experiences lay the groundwork for boundless healing, allowing for growth, transformation, and perhaps even a new form of joy.

WHAT IF MY PARTNER DOESN'T UNDERSTAND?

You may find yourself in a situation where your partner doesn't fully understand why you are grieving. While they know that you certainly endured medical trauma, they may not realize the depths to which this situation has reshaped your life. Miscarriage is absolutely a horrendous experience to have thrown at you. The emotional wounds can be so difficult to put into words that it becomes a seemingly impossible task to express what is really going on with you. Your partner's naivety on this subject may fuel new levels of isolation, frustration, anger, and rage, but all of that can be avoided through the following steps.

First, take a step back and remember that your partner is not your enemy. They are victims of miscarriage too. Although you are the one who bears the physical pain and the brunt of the emotional scars, they lost out on bringing a new life into the world just like you did. Secondly, a brief educational lesson may be in order so that they can grasp what you are in the middle of. Assume that they don't know the information you are about to give, then after your conversation, direct them to the internet so they can research on their own for more clarity. If you know the type of miscarriage that you had, tell them that. Provide your partner with how many weeks along you were. Tell them that according to the number of weeks you were, that's how long you had a life growing inside of you. They can look up visuals of fetal growth in weeks and see fruit size comparisons. Explain that your maternal instincts cause you to have strong ties to your loss and that you need to properly grieve the life that could have been. Explain that you have already envisioned your new family life, and you are also grieving the fact that you will no longer be a participant in that. Tell your partner that even though you made it to your specific number of weeks, you had already formed a bond with your baby.

Reiterate that grief has no timeline and that you will naturally move through all the stages of grief at a pace that is specific to you. Grief is an evolution of internal struggles that focuses on a despondent event. You will gain skills to cope with the event and make progress in your life. No one knows how long the process will take, but you need to extend some grace while you are still in the process. End the conversation by letting your partner know of any known triggers you have and how they make you feel when you hear or see certain things. Be sure to also stress that these triggers may change over time, and you may also have additional triggers that have yet to materialize.

CREATING A SAFE SPACE: EMOTIONAL SAFETY AT HOME

Curating an environment at home that prioritizes emotional safety creates a fortress against the disruption of grief. Within these walls, vulnerability can stretch out its roots, invited and aided with patience. Creating an emotionally safe environment turns any space into a sanctuary, producing a setting where healing can begin and flourish. Think about designating spaces within your home specifically for introspection or meditation. Let it be a place with relaxed corners where contemplation and tranquility can coexist. Here, the outside world's noise fades away, creating a peaceful environment that encourages thoughtful reflection. No grandeur is needed, and adornments can remain minimalistic yet submerged with depth. The tangible surroundings impact the emotional atmosphere. Introduce elements like soft lighting to soothe and invite tranquility, the gentle flicker of candlelight, or a warm lamp's glow imparting calm across the space. Incorporating elements like calming music draws devotion to the calming presence, each note beckoning still in an otherwise bustling world.

Invoking openness among household members fortifies safety. Encourage transparency in expressing thoughts and feelings. Conversations can be a cornerstone for crafting devotion steeped in love. Organize regular family gatherings to discuss emotional needs or tend to specific concerns, reasserting contrasts of unity and a commitment to collective well-being. The joint readying of an emotionally safe haven transforms mere shelter into a temple cherished by all.

By becoming an arena in which acceptance and common awareness thrive, home extends beyond physical boundaries to reflect an internal state of mental ease, promoting unconstrained and sincere introspection. This yields insight into the very nature of what you are going through, empowering you with toughness against life's adversities.

Though developing such spaces takes time, the rewards parallel the inherent patience and enduring dedication involved. Challenges in maintaining emotional safety may arise, particularly during difficult times, yet bearing witness to the foundational principles of compassion confirms that such a space is integral to growth and recovery. Continue confidently into the subsequent chapters of healing, embracing the importance of engagement in relationships after a loss. This integration effectuates a powerful rehearsal of connection and community, fundamental to your enduring process of recovery. Building a lasting legacy of tenderness and consciousness becomes the bedrock of your transformed future as life's experiences enrich your heart and mind.

Actionable Item: Joint Healing Activities

Explore joint activities that offer refuge and recovery for both partners. Consider these reflective questions to guide you:

- What activities, past or present, have brought both of you peace and joy?
- How can you merge these activities into your daily or weekly routine?
- Are there new practices, mindful or otherwise, you wish to explore together?

SEEKING PROFESSIONAL HELP: THERAPISTS AND SUPPORT GROUPS

Turning to professional support can emerge as a lifeline, providing you with the tools and guidance to cross insurmountable emotional landscapes. If you are experiencing persistent feelings of hopelessness, it may be time to speak to a therapist. In other words, if you consistently feel sadness more than any other emotion, it is time for you to reach out and talk with someone about that. A therapist's office becomes a haven where you can unfurl your emotions under thoughtful guidance, gaining coping skills designed to resonate with your specific circumstances.

Therapists steeped in expertise concerning grief and reproductive health ideally suit your needs, guiding discussions that address your personal context of loss. Consider credentials and experience before selection, ensuring that the therapist's expertise aligns with your situation. Don't shy away from discussing their approach because it is an integral step that helps determine their suitability for your needs. A therapist becomes an ally in assimilation, seeking to clarify processes through darkening emotions.

In addition to credentials, consider the therapeutic modalities they practice. The choice of approach may significantly impact how you heal. Embrace the opportunity to have an initial conversation with potential therapists so you can recite your story and gauge how comfortable you feel within their professional presence. It's important to feel respected, understood, and supported as you tunnel into the emotional depths of your experience with miscarriage. Therapy can be an ongoing resource, not just a tool used during times of crisis.

Schedule regular check-ins after your completion for an added layer of support.

Therapists provide footholds in processing challenging emotions, offering tools to challenge negative thought patterns. Cognitive Behavioral Therapy (CBT) is helpful in instilling healthier perspectives. It helps individuals to identify and change unhelpful thought patterns and behaviors. CBT offers a more structured and goal-oriented approach to solving problems and developing coping skills. Dialectical Behavioral Therapy (DBT) is also a healthy choice in talk therapy solutions. This evidence-based form of therapy is great for managing intense emotions. It builds upon elements of CBT by introducing Zen principles of mindfulness and compassion while simultaneously assimilating emotional regulation, acceptance, and validation. This therapeutic method can uncover new coping mechanisms that enable forward movement irrespective of blame.

Support groups offer complementary dimensions to healing by bringing together individuals united by the unfortunate experience of loss. In-person groups provide a platform for companionship and association, sharing stories punctuated by laughter and tears. In these gatherings, kindness and cohesion effortlessly weave together, forming a stronger community fabric. This collective bond serves as a powerful reminder that you are not moving through life in isolation.

Support is not just about what we receive. Giving support can be just as healing and transformative. Sharing experiences can unpack feelings and provide guidance to those in similar circumstances. These interactions influence purpose, extending the network into a wider circle of collective growth and empowerment. Explore various resources thoughtfully, selecting what aligns with your vision of healing. Therapy may resonate with some, while others find cheer in group solidarity. Your unique emotional landscape dictates your necessary environment, whether through a therapeutic space or virtual kinship.

The pursuit of well-being incorporates flexibility and an attunement to evolving emotional states. Adaptability will help synthesize the dimensions of support available, assisting spiritedness and personal growth through the process of healing. Seek professional support confidently, knowing it unlocks doors to self-discovery and renewed strength. This choice is a testament to your enduring courage and commitment, gifting you with the emboldened prospect of renewed joy. Integrating professional aid into healing habits widens your capacity for endurance, allowing you to craft meaningful transformations contrived through knowledge, compassion, and connectivity. These structured support systems intertwine to establish an enduring foundation where growth amid loss becomes possible.

ONLINE COMMUNITIES: FINDING DIGITAL SUPPORT

Modern online landscapes offer a multitude of avenues towards connection and healing, allowing those affected by miscarriage to tap into support networks that transcend geographical boundaries. Through digital platforms, individuals are afforded a new dimension of solidarity and confirmation that is discernible from the affinity of concerted experiences. Online support groups add complementary flexibility and accessibility. The faceless aspect of online platforms adds safety, encouraging individuals to express fears, aspirations, and insights without concern for recognition or credence. These platforms enable round the clock access to conversations, ensuring support even during silent, solitary nights when your grief feels most pronounced.

Social media platforms like Facebook house groups dedicated to pregnancy loss support, full of individuals passionate about expressing kindness and comprehensive discussion. Such groups feature thematic forums ranging from emotional recovery strategies to medical discussions, facilitating a warm environment rich with conjunct wisdom and insights. Platforms like Reddit's r/miscarriage grant entrance to communal halls where stories are exchanged and support extended. This specific subreddit can serve as an empathetic haven, where stories thrive in the spirit of collective benevolence. Members rally to impart guidance, encircling one another during the tribulations of miscarriage with reassurance and compassion.

These online sanctuaries render anonymity one of their greatest gifts. Individuals who seek privacy in digital spaces often find it easier to disclose deeply personal reflections or inquiries, free from social apprehensions linked to recognition. This veil empowers vulnerability, urging deeper integration among strangers united by a common thread.

Variable pitfalls can exist within the expansive digital realm. The potential for misinformation beckons caution, so take note of that with any advice received and verify it before integration when it comes to trying to heal. Protecting your mental space also requires mindfulness of interactions that evoke negativity or seem overwhelming. Online spaces warrant careful navigation to extract the highest benefit from united insights. Despite these considerations, the interconnected world of online communities stands as a formidable support stalwart, offering connection, comprehension, and goodwill to those dealing with loss. Appreciating both traditional and digital modes offers clearance for enrichment, adaptation, and harmony in healing.

Despite presenting certain challenges, digital spaces remain unequivocally invaluable for those yearning for connection while in solitude. Active involvement in these spaces transforms pain and isolation into the potential for collective healing. Merging these insights with personal reflections further enhances and authenticates the ascent to healing. Stories told in these spaces illustrate collaborative episodes, offering connection to participants dealing with similar dispositions. These interactions patronize adaptive strength, infusing ways to persevere into your emotional framework while being a testament to the collective human will to thrive.

Opportunities to contribute and offer support emerge where virtual communities proliferate. Sharing authentic experiences alleviates the internal weight and extends a virtual hand of solidarity to others. Offering guidance and goodwill implants the desire for a neighborly connection within communal spheres. Search through a variety of digital platforms, selecting spaces that resonate with your emotional cadence and comfort level. Remember, each platform extends distinctive backdrops and focal points, which warrant exploration to determine your digital retreat. Engaging meaningfully in these frontiers fabricates lasting support, ensuring that each interaction contributes subtle layers of softness and harmony to your tale of healing.

As individuals flock to these virtual domains, they learn they are not alone in their struggles. The experiences and collective strength of companions previously unknown provide raw encouragement and support. Such exchanges brighten the broader spectrum of human endurance, infusing reassurance and inspiration into each chapter of grief and things beyond. The binding lesson is that while digital platforms contain unparalleled resources, balancing them alongside offline interactions and professional guidance ensures a holistic approach. This approach significantly reinforces emotional bravery as a comprehensive structure for restoration and renewal, untethering you from the isolation of loss.

MISCARRIAGE HEARTBREAK

A FAMILY'S GUIDE TO PROCESS GRIEF, RESTORE EMOTIONAL STRENGTH, AND LEARN EFFECTIVE WAYS TO OFFER GENUINE SUPPORT AFTER PREGNANCY LOSS

"You were given this life because you are strong enough to live it."

SERENA WILLIAMS

"Grief is the price we pay for love."

QUEEN ELIZABETH II

Have you ever met someone who has had a miscarriage? Is that person a co-worker, neighbor, friend, family member, or even you? Did you pick up on their sadness and wish you could genuinely help support them through their times of grief? Perhaps you met this person well after this traumatic time in their life and you didn't know how to respond when this topic came up in conversation.

Would you take a moment to help someone who has answered yes to at least one of these questions—someone who is curious, hurting, and unsure where to begin after a miscarriage?

My hope is to make miscarriage easier to understand, and to help families feel supported and less alone. But to do that, I need your help.

Many people decide what books to read based on reviews. A simple review from you could help someone who really needs it. Your voice matters.

Leaving a review takes less than a minute. It's free, and it could change someone's life.

Your review might help...

- One more parent feel less alone
- One more family understand how to support each other
- One more caregiver feel seen

To make a difference, just scan the QR code or go to this link to leave a review:

https://www.amazon.com/review/review-your-purchases/?asin=B0F9XH549Q

Thank you from the bottom of my heart.

With love,

Tae Simeon

CHAPTER 5
ADDRESSING COMMON CONCERNS AND QUESTIONS

WHY DID THIS HAPPEN? DECIPHERING THE UNKNOWN

THE QUESTION, "WHY DID THIS HAPPEN?" casts a long shadow over those who have suffered a miscarriage, leaving a lingering ache in moments of solitude. Miscarriages can arise from many factors, often beyond our grasp or influence. Chromosomal abnormalities are the most prevalent cause, occurring arbitrarily during cell division, resulting in an embryo being unable to thrive. At times, undetected health issues such as thyroid disorders or uncontrolled diabetes can also contribute to pregnancy loss, although these conditions may evade detection without a comprehensive medical evaluation.

Uterine and cervical issues, including fibroids, an incompetent cervix, and a uterine septum, can also trigger a miscarriage. Fibroids are non-cancerous tumors found around or in the uterus and can have adverse effects on a developing fetus. An incompetent cervix refers to the premature opening of the cervix during the early stages of pregnancy, stemming from structural weakness. The cervix should only start to dilate near the end of pregnancy. A uterine septum is a congenital condition in which a wall of tissue separates space inside the uterus, thus creating two uterine cavities instead of one.

Chronic medical conditions, including diabetes, lupus, and uncontrolled high blood pressure, can also cause miscarriage. Lifestyle factors such as drug use, alcohol consumption, smoking, and malnutrition are also attributed as causes. Environmental exposure to toxins, radiation, and hazardous chemicals increases the likelihood, as does severe trauma or physical injury. The risk of miscarriage increases in women over 35 years old due to chromosomal issues.

Even with strides in medical advancements, some miscarriage causes remain shrouded in mystery, adding to the aspect of uncertainty. Accepting that not every query has a definitive answer is a distinct step in the shift to healing. It involves coming to terms with the unpredictability of human existence and recognizing that the vast expanse of medical science has its constraints. Not having an answer as to why a miscarriage occurred can be extremely frustrating, but the reality is, sometimes there will be no answer. Accepting this as the answer is exceptionally grueling, given what has just happened. A non-answer can prolong the healing process, but the good news is that eventually healing will come.

Conversations with healthcare providers are pivotal for gaining a deeper insight into one's specific circumstances. Preparing questions in advance of appointments ensures a comprehensive discussion, covering potential underlying issues or addressing concerns about multiple miscarriages. Clarity is often achieved by taking an active stance regarding one's healthcare, or at least a supportive framework is established, helping to pilot the labyrinth of unknowns. Within the inquiry of "Why did this happen?" lies an invitation to coexist with facts and ambiguity as components of healing. By recognizing our knowledge's limits and extending compassion toward ourselves and others in similar situations, we lay the groundwork for better comprehension.

Actionable Item: Preparing for Your Next Appointment

In preparation for your upcoming medical consultation, reflecting on the questions you wish to pose is worthwhile. Document them in a journal or notebook, addressing medical and emotional aspects. This practice guarantees that no topic, however small, is overlooked, promoting seamless communication and facilitating collaborative exploration of your miscarriage experience.

IS IT MY FAULT? LETTING GO OF SELF-BLAME

Miscarriage often triggers bouts of self-blame, rooted in an innate yearning for explanations. In moments of grief, one may revisit past actions, haunted by what could have been done differently. This critical inclination is exacerbated by societal whispers suggesting that pregnancy outcomes rest on an individual's shoulders. Such perceptions can create a climate where blame thrives, hammering isolation and fault. However, it's mandatory to recognize that miscarriage is seldom due to one's actions. Daily endeavors, such as exercising, lifting objects, or minor dietary choices, are not responsible for pregnancy loss. Medical backing emphasizes that these activities are not causative factors. Debunking these myths with factual evidence aids in releasing the misplaced guilt weighing heavily on one's heart.

Start the process of letting go of self-blame by acknowledging the pain. Allow yourself to become fully engulfed in whatever emotions arise, even unpleasant ones. Avoiding these feelings can prevent you from being able to release the blame. Once you have admitted the relevant emotions, seek out some education about miscarriage, and you will discover, across numerous reputable sources, that most miscarriages result from chromosomal abnormalities or natural causes. Learning this information and then accepting it can significantly reduce and hopefully eliminate irrational guilt.

The next step in the process is to talk about your experience. Saying the words out loud can be a powerful way to step out from under a dark cloud. Chat with a trusted family or friend about how you are feeling. The buildup of releasing those words can reduce the power they have over you. While you are doing that, challenge the blame. If you find yourself second guessing your actions by using language such as, "Maybe if I didn't do..." or, "I knew I should not have..." then take a step back and ask yourself if there is any factual evidence that could be found from your statements. The answer is most likely going to be "no".

Move on to embracing self-compassion and become familiar with the idea that the miscarriage was out of your control. There was nothing you could do to prevent this devastating outcome. The last step in the process is to allow yourself the time to heal. Over time, the self-blame should subside, and your broken heart can start to mend. Time really does play a significant role in the intensity of your emotions, so keep this in mind and allow things to happen organically.

FIGHTING BACK AGAINST GUILT

You may feel like your inner self critic has taken control over your rational consciousness and is on a tangent going berserk at times. There are ways to dismantle guilt when you feel this internal battle brewing. The process begins with the confession of those guilty feelings. Instead of suppressing them, admit that you know the cause of the guilt stems from the miscarriage, and move on to remind yourself to extend self-compassion. We have already reviewed the causes of miscarriage, and largely, the causes cannot be controlled. Yes, your body was the vehicle in which the baby was to develop, but that does not translate to the reason for which the undesired outcome occurred.

Express your feelings with a member or members of your support system. They will naturally assist you by providing realistic reasons to fight against guilt. Should you find yourself stuck in a perpetual loop of negative thoughts, consider being open to changing your perspective. Think about your positive qualities and forgive yourself by accepting that the miscarriage was something beyond any realistic parameters within your control.

EXPLORING SUPPORTIVE CONVERSATIONS

Creating an environment where blame is actively dismantled involves developing support networks. Engaging with support groups can be a step toward affirmative interaction. Such spaces invite individuals to be a part of the experience without sentiment, enabling collective wisdom and compassionate acceptance. Encouraging open dialogues with friends and family about emotions, especially vulnerability, can soothe the harshness of self-blame, replacing it with support and guidance.

It's perfectly fine to distance yourself from those who are not supportive because the name of the game is protecting your peace. Seek out a compassionate individual who offers a listening ear without prejudice and honors your personal boundaries. Choose your level of vulnerability to decide how much you want to share. You do not have to include every detail of your experience, only what feels doable to you. You could say something like, "I had a miscarriage and it's affecting me more than I expected. Can I tell you something?" or "I went through something rough very recently and I'm not sure how to talk about it, but I want to try."

Supportive conversations are dual sided and conversational prompts can be used to invite genuine connection. If you are the support person for someone who has just experienced a miscarriage, there is dialogue that you can engage with for meaningful assistance. Examples would be, "Can we talk about what support looks like for you right now?", or "What is something that made you feel seen during a hard time?", or "What has helped you when you felt lost or disconnected?" Partner-specific language could be, "What helps you feel close to me," and "Can we talk about how this has changed us and what we are learning?"

Sometimes, words are hard to express, so an emotional bridge is needed to get to the other side of grief. Ways to cross a bridge would be to send a text or forward a social media post that resonates. There are endless examples online to convey the message you want to get across, so take your time and choose a message that fits the situation.

HOW TO TALK TO CHILDREN ABOUT MISCARRIAGE

Conversations about miscarriage with children often necessitate a delicate blend of honesty and sensitivity. Children are intuitive and absorb the emotional environment around them. They benefit from truthful yet age-appropriate discussions that make complicated concepts digestible without overwhelming them. Simple language can offer clarity. An example might be: "The baby was too small to keep growing in Mommy's tummy."

To ensure effective communication, align your message with the child's developmental stage. Their age and emotional maturity may dictate how the conversation is led. Younger children often follow along through stories, which can help them visualize complicated concepts. You could liken the situation to a flower that needed more sunshine to flourish. For older kids, direct, honest dialogue is preferable. You could be a bit more detailed and use clear language to build emotional clarity and trust. Encouraging questions prompt trust and provide a safe space for them to make sense of the situation. No matter how you choose to handle this conversation, be sure to create a safe space for the little ones and reassure them that this is not their fault (or yours).

As children process loss, know that they too may grieve. Be receptive to their expressions, whether through dialogue, drawing, or play. Reassure them that it's okay to feel sadness or confusion and that love within the family is unyielding. This emotional support is a prerequisite for helping them navigate their own feelings and reinforce the security of the family structure.

Including children in remembrance rituals can be therapeutic for everyone involved. A family memory book can serve as a tangible keepsake, where children contribute art or thoughts, cementing precious memories within its pages. Alternatively, a memorial garden planted together can symbolize cycles of life and revitalization. Watching the garden bloom stands as an organic reminder of life's continuation. These activities bestow a sense of contribution and comprehension, helping children perceive love's unwavering nature in the presence of loss.

DEVELOPING EMOTIONAL UNDERSTANDING

Building emotional intelligence in children involves ongoing dialogue about loss and healing. Introducing stories with themes of resilience and recovery can deepen their appreciation of emotions. Literature that explores diverse experiences of grief helps demystify the concept. Encouraging reflective discussions around these stories enriches children's emotional vocabulary and aids them in figuring out their internal worlds.

Check in with your own emotions before conversing with children regarding developing their emotional understanding. If you are carrying grief, confusion, or fear, be cognizant of that. Maintaining awareness of your own emotional state can help you remain calm and present during the conversations. This is key since children have a knack for knowing when something is wrong, as they can sense tension or sadness without even knowing the specifics. It is your job to validate their feelings and reinforce security, even though they may not be aware of what is happening. Encourage ongoing conversations to assist in their development and take it a step further by modeling what healthy grief looks like. Healthy grief is present when you prove that you have free flowing emotions by showing that it is okay to cry or speak about difficult subjects. Being open with your feelings and showing that hiding your feelings is unnecessary will help tackle this task.

Interactive Element: Creating Your Family Memory Book

Gather relevant items like photos or keepsakes to establish a family memory book. Prompt family members, children included, to contribute something personally meaningful. Set aside time regularly to add entries or reflect on existing ones. This ongoing project preserves your history and strengthens familial bonds through collective healing and remembrance. Empathetic and thoughtful dialogues aid children in processing loss healthily, shaping a foundation of honesty and support. Their comprehension evolves with age, but the honesty you impart now will carry them through future adversities with gallantry and compassion.

CREATING MEMORIES: HONORING YOUR LOSS

Instituting rituals to memorialize loss provides structured opportunities for transformation through meaningful actions, paying homage to both past experiences and present existence. Observing a ritual, such as lighting a candle on significant dates, be it an anniversary or a day of loss, becomes symbolic. The glow's warmth and the time are marked for reflection, each flickering flame a testament to remembrance, bonding individual and collective expression.

When considering rituals that honor, personalize activities that symbolically carry forward a legacy of continued existence. A custom engraved stone or a beautiful garden statue can be created and placed in a meaningful location to honor a loss. Crafting a memory box enclosing treasured mementos like photos, letters, and keepsakes builds a private record only you comprehend. Personalizing memories like custom jewelry, stuffed animals, or blankets permits the continuity of love, crisscrossing its legacy through tangible exchanges treasured over time.

Gathering for communal rituals offers collective healing rooted in strength and remembered joy. Putting together intimate gatherings unites individuals bound by connection through loss, forging a space for synergistic healing. Within this collective embrace, spoken and silent bonds draw on past memories while sowing seeds of a favorable outlook. Each personalized act of remembrance stands as a celebration of love, embodying the imprint of lives touched and the enduring influence of cherished legacies. Embracing these expressions ripens healing practices, yielding the present's continuity despite past loss through lovingly upheld rituals.

Another way to honor your loss is through permanent body art in the form of a tattoo. Tattooing as a therapeutic ritual varies in symbolism, yet universally transforms grief into a powerful visual testament. Getting a tattoo can involve some pain for most people, especially depending on the body part being tattooed. Mindfulness and endurance are two practices that go along with the process, so those benefits will be present.

Getting tattooed in a spot where you can see it without needing a mirror can serve to transform your emotional scars and reclaim control. This form of expression can be unique to you, or you can choose well-known miscarriage imagery such as two birds on a perch with the third flying away, angel wings with one date, or a miscarriage and pregnancy loss ribbon. I chose to get my right leg tattooed with a very large winding stem with leaves, two of which have my miscarriage dates on them. People within the tattoo community get their ink for a variety of reasons, and miscarriage tattoos are commonplace today. A cathartic expression of love such as this creates a safe and tangible way to communicate grief while it reflects on a life that was lost. Once the tattoo is finished, you will be left with beautiful body art to admire and a way to memorialize the loss permanently.

EXPLORING FUTURE PREGNANCY OPTIONS: INFORMED DECISIONS

Deciding to pursue another pregnancy after a miscarriage demands thoughtful deliberation, medically and emotionally. Initial steps often involve a thorough medical examination. Engaging with a fertility specialist can highlight personal circumstances and uncover underlying factors contributing to prior loss. Genetic counseling may be advised, especially if recurrent miscarriages have occurred, revealing any genetic linkages that might affect future pregnancies, and providing clarity to make informed decisions.

Emotional readiness is just as important as physical health when contemplating another pregnancy. Assessing your emotional state and your willingness to embark on this territory again is critical. Engage in open conversations with your significant other to align emotional readiness and amplify dual assimilation. Both partners have experienced the loss, so this concept must not be one-sided. The depths of emotions that coincide with miscarriage can vary from one person to another, so it is all-important that both parties be truthful and in agreement on where their mental health stands. These dialogues reinforce dedication to face the road ahead, reinforcing your relationship's strength.

Medical advancements continue to introduce new methods to support future pregnancies. Progesterone supplements, for example, might be recommended as a preventive strategy in the case of a history of miscarriage. These supplements help preserve a pregnancy by supporting the uterine lining, minimizing the risk of early loss. With a personalized care plan, these innovations instill encouragement and reassurance.

A continual open dialogue with healthcare providers remains major throughout. Preparing for preconception counseling sessions with predefined questions or concerns enriches these discussions. Include topics like potential treatments, lifestyle changes, or any other worries regarding conceiving. This proactive method enriches your relationship with healthcare and compliments a collaborative relationship with your medical team, ensuring tailored support in every corner.

In planning a future pregnancy, intertwining medical insight with emotional conscience formulates a cohesive plan. Each step, from specialist consultations to heartfelt home dialogues, reinforces a base of informed choices and mutual comprehension. The approach requires a commitment to a potential new life and the holistic well-being of all individuals involved.

REGULATING EMOTIONAL LANDSCAPES

Your emotional landscape before pursuing another pregnancy can be nuanced. Reflecting on past experiences with mindfulness and counseling aids in processing residual emotions. Ask yourself meaningful open-ended questions to gear up for introspection, assisting in establishing emotional readiness. The line of questioning can focus on inquiring about your own core values, exploring how your actions align with your values, how you respond to stress, and any progress you have made towards your long-term goals. Supplement self-awareness and practice gratitude by honing in on positive aspects of your life, including your surrounding loved ones.

Taking a moment to confess your strengths and weaknesses honestly will open the door for you to give yourself some grace. Additionally, second level thinking will allow you to avoid jumping to conclusions so that you can consider alternative explanations. These practices support emotional exploration, granting clarity to pursue future parenthood with a composed mind.

ADDRESSING THE FEAR OF CONCEIVING AGAIN

Fear often takes root after miscarriage, serving as a protector against the unknown. It symbolizes a defense mechanism, shielding from possible heartache. Decoding this fear is obligatory. It's not indicative of weakness, but a natural response to past loss. Many women find themselves caught between a wish and fear, questioning if their maternal dreams could come to fruition. This fear, though mighty, mustn't govern you. Recognizing it forms part of your emotional landscape and is a step towards its management.

Coping strategies can soothe this anxiety, providing relief during times of uncertainty. Find things that can calm the mind and provide an outlet for anxiety to turn fear into creativity. Professional therapy sessions offer another option, creating an impartial zone where fears can be vocalized and managed. Therapy serves to untangle involuted emotions, supporting perseverance.

Support systems take an instrumental role in alleviating fears. Discussing anxieties with a partner invites applicable fathoming and understanding. These conversations don't need immediate solutions. Their impact lies in the admission of emotions. Trusted friends offer comfort, reminding you that you are surrounded by caring people. Their congenial words can serve as a binder in moments of doubt.

Setting sights on positive outcomes helps develop optimism for the future. Reading stories of successful pregnancies following loss inspires courage. These portrayals illustrate the possibility beyond fear, teaching that while past experiences mold you, they don't wholly dictate your future. Support groups are replete with such stories, forming a community abundant with mass triumph. Engaging with these communities endorses an environment of belonging.

CHIPPING AWAY AT UNCERTAINTY: ACCEPTING THE UNKNOWNS OF FUTURE ATTEMPTS

The future is unknown to us all, so embrace uncertainty. Have a discussion with your partner to discuss the inevitability of uncertainty in future pregnancies and how to embrace it. Remember, you are not in full control when it comes to pregnancy, so don't worry about things you cannot control or change. Instead, take charge of what you can control.

You can do this by being mindful of how you treat your body, how you build emotional support, how you achieve resilience, and how you are open to all possible outcomes. You can balance hope and reality by believing in a statement like, "I'm hopeful, although I know the outcome is something I can't control." This is how dreams and caution can coexist. Keep your focus on the things in the present and miles away from "what if" statements. The hypothetical line of thinking can cause emotional spirals and induce unnecessary anxiety.

DECIDING TO STOP TRYING: FINDING PEACE WITH THE DECISION

The recognition of personal limits is serious. It is up to you to be aware of personal limits and know when enough is enough. Emotional and physical indicators of exhaustion will confirm this for you. You will need to be at peace with and accept the decision to stop trying. Some couples have the misfortune of experiencing several miscarriages before they choose to end the attempts. That level of trauma can be damaging to the core.

Deciding to forgo future pregnancy attempts should exhaust all avenues before coming to a complete stop. Both partners need to be equally involved in this decision. There are options available should a couple decide that they absolutely cannot handle an additional pregnancy. The male could undergo a vasectomy, which is a safe and effective surgical procedure for male birth control. Alternatively, the female could undergo a tubal ligation, which is a safe and effective surgical procedure that prevents pregnancy in women. Mental health in good standing is highly recommended before exercising one of these invasive and permanent procedures. Ensure there are no doubts about moving forward with one of these procedures to remove any room for future expressions of regret.

Personally, I chose to undergo a procedure called a bilateral salpingectomy a couple of months after my second miscarriage. This is a permanent form of birth control in which both fallopian tubes are removed, and it also reduces the risk of ovarian cancer. My husband and I discussed permanent birth control options at length in the months leading up to my final pregnancy, and I knew I was going to move forward with that regardless of whatever happened after that pregnancy. Although I was confident with my choice to have this procedure before my last pregnancy, during the pregnancy, and even on the day of surgery, I developed some level of regret months later when I suddenly seemed to be bombarded with triggers. I second guessed my decision big time. Pregnancy announcements were popping up from various people all over my social media feeds, so I had to unplug for a while. I relied on distractions like taking pictures and videos of my dog and working extra hours at my job to keep my mind busy. Before I knew it, I had once again made peace with the decision. I had never contemplated that I would face regret regarding this type of decision. It was well thought out and planned in advance in my mind, given how traumatic an experience I had with the first miscarriage. I knew deep down that I could not risk having a third miscarriage because I was already mentally depleted after the first one. To date, the first one still haunts me, but I'm no longer allowing it to define me.

Engaging in therapy can help you process any decision you make and the subsequent emotions. Celebrate new beginnings and opportunities that arise from this decision. Alternative options for parenthood are highly encouraged, including adoption and fostering. When and if you are ready and able, begin researching adoption agencies and the processes followed to allow you to bring a child into your home. Children of all ages need loving homes, and they are located in every part of the world. This may be the answer for your family if you are unable to maintain a viable pregnancy.

DIVERSE PERSPECTIVES: CULTURAL HANDLING OF MISCARRIAGES

The ways in which different cultures perceive and process miscarriage contribute to a diverse mosaic of traditions and attitudes. This variety shapes the unique approaches individuals take in dealing with loss. Women largely carry the emotional load, and their fertility is strongly connected to their social identity. It is common for the silence and stigma of miscarriage to intensify feelings of isolation, as public mourning is often discouraged.

Numerous African traditions use rituals where herbal womb cleansing ceremonies serve as organic support mechanisms. A common theme across African culture is that miscarriage is tied to ancestors or spirits, instead of it being a medical travesty. It is believed that miscarriage is a result of ancestral intervention stemming from either protection or unresolved ancestral issues. Some see miscarriage as a spiritual imbalance or a curse. For instance, in West Africa, miscarriage has a spiritual framing that is linked to the metaphysical world. They refer to a cycle of death and rebirth as "abiku", a spirit child who was never meant to stay. The child was born to die and repeatedly be reborn to torment the mother. Special rituals are performed by traditional healers to determine the spiritual cause and convince the rebirth spirit to stay, ensuring the ancestors and/or deities are pleased. In East Africa, rituals may be performed to cleanse the body and household. Prayer, fasting, and community support may play a role in healing here. Depending on gestational age, the fetus may not be named or formally buried. There is a stigma involved in which the mother may be viewed as unlucky and even to blame if she has suffered multiple losses.

Certain Asian traditions emphasize internal reflection, viewing silence as a dual homage of respect and personal grief respite. There are parts of Asian culture where ceremonies are held featuring small statues, and families can present gifts and pray to help the family cope with loss. In Japan, a memorial service known as a Mizuko Kuyo is held at a temple to honor a lost child. Incense are lit and toys, flowers, or clothing is offered. This private and spiritual service is a way to release grief in a neutral way. In China, miscarriage is sometimes viewed as an imbalance of yin and yang. It is believed that the fetus's spirit can linger and affect future fertility or health. Some women choose to follow zuo yuezi, which translates to a month of rest, warmth, and recovery. Acupuncture, herbal soups, and a particular diet are used to induce physical and spiritual healing. Public mourning is also largely frowned upon in China, which again brings the stigma and shame to the mother.

Cultural context wields substantial influence over grieving. In some societies, stigma and silence surrounding miscarriages are prevalent, creating barriers to open mourning. This cultural decorum can intensify feelings of seclusion, as customary expectations can deter public declaration of grief.

Meanwhile, in many Latin American cultures, an extensive family network often forms an integral support network. Family members band together to offer both practical and emotional backing during the mourning period. Celebrations known as Día de los Muertos, or the Day of the Dead, celebrate deceased loved ones, with miscarried babies being honored on November 1st during Día de los Angelitos, or Day of the Little Angels.

Support mechanisms in various cultures present unique healing styles. Seeking counsel from traditional healers or spiritual guides is typical in societies where spirituality is esteemed. Their presence can soothe, serving as a liaison between the physical and metaphysical realms. Commemorative gatherings to honor the departed also add to healing, facilitating structured grieving. Such gatherings promote storytelling, where sharing experiences becomes transformative for communal healing.

Personal stories reveal levels of tenacity in those experiencing miscarriage. A woman might transform adversity into advocacy, using her experiences to aid others in similar trials. Another might find peace in artistic expression, where creations communicate unvoiced emotions. This diversity underscores how personal growth often arises from adversity, enkindling favor and familiarity with others who have traversed similar challenges.

For some, faith and spirituality establish a navigation framework through loss. Religious practices offer stillness through prayer or meditation, a channel where grief unites with a higher power. However, faith also presents challenges. Pondering why suffering occurs can stir internal discord.

Reconciling belief with loss involves reflection and occasionally reevaluating one's faith.

EMBRACING DIVERSE GRIEF PROCESSES

Honoring diverse grief processes includes embracing global perspectives and practices. This open mindedness allows integration of different cultural healing mechanisms. It entails respecting distinct grieving conventions while drawing meaningful elements into your own healing story. Participating in cross-cultural exchanges broadens our comprehension and presents novel solutions to dealing with grief on a global scale. Grieving the loss of someone can look different from person to person. Some people may find comfort in prayers, rituals, or traditions, but others may not want to explore those routes. Find something that speaks to you and take your time.

PERSONAL NARRATIVES: VOICES OF STRENGTH AND RESILIENCE

During deep loss, personal tales emerge as symbols of tenacity. Take, for instance, a woman whom we will refer to as Mariah. Mariah has experienced five miscarriages in her lifetime, all between weeks 10 and 17 of pregnancy. She has no living children. Despite overwhelming grief, Mariah discovered a renewed sense of purpose in advocacy. She developed a supportive network for similarly affected individuals and transformed herself out of desolation into someone who became a champion of change. Her actions uplifted herself and countless others, highlighting how adversity forges deeply compassionate action. Her transition from despair to hope underscores how sharing her experiences could shed light on pathways for others, crafting a community grounded in reasoning and kindness.

Now, let's look at Shannon's story. Shannon is in her early thirties and has four sisters, all of whom have young children. She is very active in their lives. Shannon is also an elementary school teacher, so her world revolves around kids. Shannon was excited to welcome her first child, but suffered a miscarriage during week 14 of her pregnancy. She had already begun to show and had started telling people about her blossoming bundle of joy. Faced with bouts of chronic depression, she couldn't bear returning to work in such a child-focused environment. Nonstop triggers became too much for her, so she left her profession and turned to bartending to escape her surroundings. Over time, she developed a rapport with repeat patrons, and some of them began telling her their personal stories of triumph after miscarriage. She was encouraged to join one of their online support groups, which she did, and credits that for giving her the strength to return to early childhood education, which was her true love. Shannon is an example of how stepping away from something for a while can be beneficial in allowing your heart to heal.

Finally, we look at Diego. He and his wife of 8 years had been trying to start a family for years, but they have unfortunately experienced three miscarriages, all between 8 and 10 weeks. Diego's wife, Corina, had seemingly healed mentally from the losses, but Diego still struggled, even years later. He desperately wanted to become a father, as all his male friends and immediate family members were. He had experienced outside pressure suggesting that he leave his wife for someone who could bear and carry children, but he honored his vows and loved his wife too deeply to disappoint her in that way. Facing enormous pressure from seemingly everyone except his wife, Diego set up and attended grief counseling. He attended multiple sessions alone, and his wife joined him in the final two sessions. They discussed family planning options but did not agree on alternative ways to bring a child into the home, as Corina wanted to leave the door open to a natural, viable pregnancy. She felt that she was mentally strong enough to endure additional losses should they occur. She believed they would be rewarded with children when the time was right. Almost a year after the last counseling session, Corina and Diego welcomed their first child into the world, a healthy 8lb baby boy, born full term. In their case, they needed more time. The birth of their son taught them resilience, and Diego was able to end his grief over yearning to become a father, although he will never forget about the previous losses.

Adversity prompts unexpected growth. Those who have crawled through loss's maze develop a keener perspective on grasping nuances within others' struggles. This maturation enriches interpersonal attachments, deepening bonds with loved ones and strangers. The lesson of mortality encourages reflection on the delicate nature of life and the moments we hold dear. From this perspective, individuals discover strength in surviving and thriving.

These stories can inspire you to see that a favorable future with ideal outcomes can be achieved. They decide how adversity can be the foundation for miracles, often where we least expect them. By sharing these narratives, we find solidarity in human experience and recognition that strength can be achieved in numerous forms.

HONORING STORYTELLING'S TRANSFORMATIVE POWER

Recognizing storytelling's transformative power means engaging with statement sharing beyond personal experiences. Its potency lies in binding individual threads into a collective unit of experiences. When community members decide to talk about their experiences, know that they are authentic in their feelings and voices. Platforms dedicated to these stories facilitate healing and community building. Whether narrating stories through memoirs or blogs, sharing invites others into intimate vulnerability spaces. These accounts break isolation barriers, transmitting solidarity to the audience. They help to make sense of the pain and reveal change. The wisdom poured into these stories comes from a source that has walked the same path as you at some point. As stories travel, they generate drips of transformation, dismantling stigma, and advocating for environments that honor and amplify diverse sentiments.

Urging others to open up about their history multiplies this impact, forming a symphony of authentic and courageous voices. These dedicated platforms become sanctuaries where stories resonate with passion and courage. Every story becomes bound to the next within this space, transcending singular experience. Story sharing becomes a precious gift exchange, honoring the storyteller and the listener with honesty's raw humanity.

THE ROLE OF ART AND CREATIVITY IN PROCESSING GRIEF

Art and creativity offer therapeutic outlets for articulating grief. Emotions emerge that words struggle to convey. Artistic engagement allows emotional exploration through tangible methods. Painting or drawing becomes a therapeutic release, converting inexplicable feelings into visual expressions. Each line or shape embodies emotion, reformulating inner turbulence into a visual dialogue. Through art, the subtleties of thought and emotion find clarity and voice.

Countless individuals find security in art, transforming it into an emotional bridge. Take those crafting murals in memory of lost pregnancies. These vibrant artworks become a communal tribute to loss, morphing personal sorrows into collective divulgence. Art creation is therapeutic, aiding in sewing together life's fragmented pieces into something meaningful. Projects like these resonate well beyond personal healing; they craft dialogue, serve as community bridges, and inspire connection.

Creative communities magnify the way towards healing. Workshops or artistic groups provide conducive environments for sharing stories to construct support. Community art projects allow bonding with others on a similar trajectory, creating consensual encouragement and inspiration. Within these groups, collective creation forms a language, bridging gaps within individual experiences and encouraging connectivity.

Starting with a personal art portfolio benefits newcomers eager to explore artistic possibilities. This private venue permits unfiltered, spontaneous expression and grappling with grief through sketches, colors, or writing. Participating in art therapy sessions facilitates structured creative exploration under a therapist's guidance, which devises a secure, exploratory space for emotions.

Overall, art and creativity pose powerful mechanisms for processing grief, breaking boundaries, and unlocking learning opportunities about oneself. Embracing creative expressions introduces new comprehension and affinities, both individually and communally.

EXPANDING ARTISTIC HEALING MEDIA

Exploring various artistic media expands the scope for emotional expression. The goal is to look for something to give your emotions a voice. Start with what feels safe before you move out of your comfort zone. Visual arts can offer one convention, while songwriting, dance, or sculpture present other unique exploration avenues. Sensory-based art, including working with clay or ceramics, and even fabric arts like quilting or embroidery, may be an enjoyable option for anyone wanting a more low-key experience.

Consider the idea that some things can be left unfinished. Leaving some pieces open can express unresolved emotions you may be carrying. Perhaps leave a design slightly unfinished or leave a drawing open for further interpretation. Experimenting with different media invites holistic healing and encourages discovering joy across creative spectrums. This unfolds both personal discovery and communal unification, contributing to the richness of creative exploration.

Actionable Item: Self-Compassion Exercise

Allocate a moment for introspection. Sit quietly, close your eyes, and place a hand over your heart. Breathe deeply, using each breath to make room for compassion within you. As you breathe, repeat affirmations that resonate with your emotional state, letting those phrases wash over you like a gentle wave, easing harsh decrees you hold against yourself. This exercise serves as a moving reminder of your worthiness for grace. In pursuing release from self-blame, recognize that healing doesn't always follow a simple sequence. Grant yourself the grace of time to truly embrace self-compassion.

CHAPTER 6
MANAGING RELATIONSHIPS AFTER LOSS

STRENGTHENING YOUR RELATIONSHIP AFTER A MISCARRIAGE

WHEN FACING the aftermath of a miscarriage, it is natural to concentrate on the personal process of mending a broken heart. However, this sorrow often extends beyond the individual, casting long shadows over relationships once tempered by love. The valleys of grief can expose hidden fissures, challenging the steadiest of bonds and revealing emotions that have long been shelved. In these delicate times, partners may find themselves adrift in a sea of emotions, unable to untangle the ostentatious knots of their grief. This personal retreat into sorrow can lead to emotional chasms between partners, as mix-ups abound, and interpreting each other's needs becomes a task fraught with wonder. One may seek appeasement in quiet, while the other yearns for dialogue, causing tension in a once harmonious bond.

Open communication is a life raft in these wild waters, guiding partners toward interconnected comprehension and renewed respect. Establishing "emotional check-ins" is critical. This can be defined as times set aside without interruptions, where partners can freely express their feelings. Simple "I feel" statements enable honesty without hostility, such as "I feel overwhelmed today." These exchanges encourage clarity, diminish defensiveness, and materialize emotional transparency. Give your full attention to your partner, pick up on their expressions, and respond thoughtfully. This ensures that both individuals feel appreciated and recognized, creating a peaceful environment conducive to empathy and respect.

Reconnecting emotionally after such a loss requires intentionality, patience, and willingness to be vulnerable. Activities inspire closeness and help reconstruct the emotional bridge, marred by heartbreak. Consider activities where you can rediscover joy together, whether in going for peaceful walks, cooking new recipes, or taking up a hobby that integrates creativity and cooperation. Such experiences reignite bonds, inviting moments of unity obscured by grief. Additionally, couples therapy can be an all-important tool for rebuilding trust and comprehension. Professional support provides a neutral platform where both can freely explore their feelings publicly while learning to inspire one another. These sessions can improve communication, expose underlying issues, and create a guide to map out a healing plan that both can undertake with renewed expectancy.

Throughout this process, patience is of great importance. Recognize that everyone grieves differently and that both personal reflection and mourning are indispensable parts of the puzzle. Emotional reactions, though diverse, are valid expressions of one's experience, deserving of validation. Validation doesn't necessitate agreement but rather a revelation of the emotions in play and respect for their existence. Strive to see the world through your partner's emotional vantage point to fortify supportive partnerships, even when diverging emotional landscapes emerge.

Despite the daunting challenges of miscarriage in a relationship, it can also serve as a crucible for growth, engendering deeper connection and potency. By handling these trials together with intentionality and compassion, partners can emerge with a stronger bond, a testament to enduring love's potential to weather and transcend grief.

Actionable Item: Emotional Check-In Journal

To complement these practices, consider maintaining an "Emotional Check-In Journal" as a tangible means to track your thoughts, feelings, and the progress of relationship dynamics over time. After check-in sessions, jot down pertinent discussion points and gain insights, reflecting on how these exchanges affect your communication patterns and emotional responses. This reflective exercise can provide clarity over time, revealing the relationship's evolution and depth of understanding. Use the journal to narrate instances of connection, misreading, and resolutions, allowing you to observe growth and patterns in your interactions.

FRIENDS AND SOCIAL CIRCLES: MAINTAINING CONNECTIONS

Enduring a miscarriage can send ripples through one's social life, altering friendships and reshaping interactions in unforeseen ways. Friends may find themselves unsure of how to approach or support you, which can enhance feelings of isolation in your grief. There may be moments when friends, normally well-meaning, avoid the topic entirely, fearing their attempts at comfort may inadvertently wound further. Likewise, invitations and conversations may shift, as friends wrestle with how to include you in social events that could be emotionally triggering. Such relations often present as a secondary loss, amplifying loneliness during an already vulnerable time.

Plugging into relationships during this period demands a nuanced balance of communication and patience. When able, consider reaching out to trusted friends, even if just for a brief, lighthearted interaction. By expressing either a willingness to discuss your experiences or calmly indicating when you prefer not to, you are laying the groundwork for future exchanges. Honesty is integral in these dealings, allowing you to communicate what genuinely aids your healing. Should certain topics or gestures be painful, establish those boundaries kindly but explicitly. True friends who value you will appreciate this transparency and strive to respect your needs, building a foundation for strengthening the relationship.

Establishing clear boundaries within your social circle is a priority for safeguarding your emotional well-being. Informing friends about topics to avoid or suggesting alternative activities that provide comfort is one of the methods to secure emotional well-being. This could mean opting for a quiet coffee chat rather than a larger social gathering. Prioritizing interactions that contribute to safety over those that provoke stress is needed. It's entirely acceptable to pull back from overwhelming social obligations, allowing for the space necessary for introspection and healing.

Friendships thrive on the principle of harmonious support, a tenet that bears greater significance in times of tribulation.

While it's important to seek support, returning it can be equally restorative. Partake in acts of kindness, such as sending an encouraging note or offering a homemade meal. These heartfelt gestures fortify your bonds and demonstrate that these relationships are grounded in an intersected understanding. By opening up about your experience, you encourage friends to explore their own struggles, developing a cycle of collective support that elaborates on healing.

Interactive Element: Friendship Reflection Exercise

Engage in a friendship reflection exercise. List the friends who have stood as flag bearers of support during this time. Next to each name, identify specific actions you can take in advancement. This exercise can punctuate the relationships that warrant investment and how best to grow them. As these lists develop, notice patterns of support and areas where more transparency or boundary setting may be beneficial. By intentionally conditioning these friendships, you manufacture a robust network of support.

Maintaining friendships after a miscarriage inevitably poses challenges, yet with honest communication and well-defined boundaries, these relationships can transform into sources of strength and repose. Engaging actively with your social circle reinforces a network of comprehension and support, shoring you up during this trying chapter of your life.

DEALING WITH PREGNANT FRIENDS AND FAMILY

The interaction with pregnant friends and family can evoke a complicated maelstrom of emotions that might be tricky to untangle. It's perfectly natural to encounter flashes of envy when facing growing bellies or hearing animated discussions about nurseries and baby names. These conversations might serve as sharp reminders of what could have been, overshadowing interactions that were once unencumbered and enjoyable. Sentiments of sadness or detachment might creep in, leaving you emotionally exhausted after these meetings. Such reactions are natural and valid, yet they can introduce intricacies into your relationships, making interactions with expectant loved ones even more convoluted.

I did not experience envious feelings when I dealt with pregnant friends and family. I was genuinely happy for their pregnancies and celebrated them. At the same time, I was heartbroken for myself, and that is where the tears came from. I had recurring flashbacks of suffering from the medical trauma of miscarriage, and it included vivid scenes of me sitting on hospital beds crying for hours. To make matters worse, this ordeal took place during the global Coronavirus pandemic, so hospitals were not allowing patients to have any guests or support people with them. Various members of the healthcare team rubbed my back and offered what they thought would be consoling words. In short, that emotional struggle between balancing happiness for others and dismembering sadness for myself pushed me into a deeper hole of anxiety and depression induced isolation. Talk about exhausting!

Governing interactions necessitates a balanced approach of self-awareness and self-care. I wish I had known this at the height of my struggle, but here I am to tell you. To protect your emotional well-being, limit your exposure to scenarios that spark intense feelings. For example, if a family function looms overwhelming, consider attending briefly or sending your regards sincerely. Prioritizing emotional health over compulsory social appearances is not only permissible but also needed. Developing self-compassion includes accepting the need to step back from situations destabilizing your emotions without guilt or needing justification.

Managing relations with pregnant friends and family may initially seem daunting or obligatory, but they don't have to become overwhelming. Proactively setting clear boundaries and engaging in respectful dialogue generates an atmosphere amenable to healing a web of ornate emotions. Empower yourself to dictate how and when to engage with these social dimensions, prioritizing interactions that cherish and uplift your healing process. Open, honest exchanges can ease the emotional strain of these interactions. Where appropriate, express your feelings to expecting friends or relatives. Communicate despite genuinely sharing in their joy, certain aspects remain taxing for you. This transparency can help avoid contention. Although not all may respond adeptly, those who are sincere will try to accommodate your needs considerately.

Maintaining self-care rituals around these encounters is imperative. Grounding techniques, including deep breathing exercises or mentally envisioning serene landscapes, can stabilize emotions during and after such exchanges. After particularly challenging interactions, consider taking time for personal replenishment by connecting with the natural world or indulging in creative activities. These practices offer mean-ingful interludes that underscore the priority of safeguarding your emotional health, far from selfish but central to healing.

Each step in managing these partnerships underscores that you can and will return to your "normal" self or an even better version. It tests many things, including discerning what aligns with your well-being, revealing the hardships involved, seeking beneficial support, and granting yourself the liberty to withdraw when needed. In so doing, you honor your grief and healing potential, creating a guided space for compassion.

Managing relationships with pregnant friends and family ultimately involves mastering the delicate teamwork of emotions and connections. It balances between respecting your feelings and keeping communication secure and supportive. As you progress, remember your needs are valid, and prioritizing them is a robust emblem of self-love.

WORKPLACE DYNAMICS: ADDRESSING PROFESSIONAL LIFE

Enduring a miscarriage impacts various aspects of life, including the professional sphere, where personal experiences may overlap with professional responsibilities. Addressing a sensitive issue after a loss poses distinctive challenges, such as contemplating how much of this personal history to reveal to colleagues or supervisors. You may feel uneasy about disclosing such an intimate experience within a professional setting, fearing potential changes in perception or uncomfortable interactions, adding to your emotional cargo. Conversely, not sharing might engender disputes regarding shifts in work performance or demeanor. Balancing transparency and privacy is shaped by your comfort within the workplace culture.

When contemplating whether to discuss your miscarriage experience at work, reflect on your workplace's capacity for support and your rapport with colleagues or supervisors. Work environments that embrace personal transparency with support can be invaluable, offering much needed accommodation. However, discretion might be wise in less sympathetic cultures or where privacy seems better protected. Restrict disclosure to critical information concerning immediate work obligations. Consider these aspects against personal preferences and weigh the potential advantages of frank communication, possibly leading to critical backing and support during recovery.

Managing work related stress while healing from a miscarriage also involves recognizing your limitations and advocating for what you need. Seeking flexible work arrangements or temporary time off can be beneficial if you feel unprepared to resume complete duties. Many workplaces offer Employee Assistance Programs (EAPs) that provide counseling services. Applying these resources can help alleviate emotional weight, allowing focus on personal healing alongside professional responsibilities. Temporarily adjusting workloads or delegating tasks when feasible can smooth the transition back to your full role.

Transitioning back to the workplace after a miscarriage requires well planned support. Taking a graduated approach in resuming responsibilities can mitigate feeling overwhelmed, permitting needed time for adjustment. Converse with HR or management regarding any accommodation you might require, such as adjusted hours or work assignments, to ease this transition. Furthermore, communicate with key colleagues about your return plan, encouraging their support in your return. This forward approach paves the way for a less stressful return to the workplace.

While contemplating whether to disclose your miscarriage at work, ponder its broader impact on professional relationships and accountability. Sharing such personal aspects in a professional place can bring about warm-heartedness and open possibilities for meaningful support. Alternatively, if you decide against disclosure, ensure there are external support systems to help direct any emerging work stressors.

Ultimately, adapting to professional life following a miscarriage involves a fine balance of transparency alongside considerations of privacy. It requires knowing your limits and confidently asserting your needs in alignment with your workplace environment. Whether sharing your experience or keeping it private, remember that self-care remains primary during this recovery period. Such decisions should optimally reflect your immediate needs, broader professional goals, and personal recuperation.

Strengthening workplace relationships during this period is invaluable. Leaning on trusted colleagues who comprehend your situation supplies additional emotional scaffolding within the professional setting. These connections confirm that handling personal setbacks and professional duties after a loss need not occur in isolation. In recognizing how miscarriage affects different life domains, including work, you empower yourself to make well informed decisions on engaging with these dynamics, consistently placing personal healing at the forefront.

Actionable Item: Reflecting on Workplace Interactions

Take a moment to reflect on your professional interactions and consider keeping a workplace journal. Document any interactions or accommodations that have been helpful, and note areas where further support might be needed. This practice can act as both a roadmap for upcoming dialogues and a reflective chronicle of your professional history affiliated with personal recovery.

REBUILDING INTIMACY: EMOTIONAL AND PHYSICAL CONNECTION

Intimacy often undergoes considerable transformation after a miscarriage, leaving couples contending with a multitude of emotions. The shadow of loss affects both the physical and emotional aspects of connection, altering a landscape once familiar and reassuring. The comfort found in linked experiences may now be overshadowed by hesitancy, as individuals deal with heartaches, dimming their desires. The fear of vulnerability, coupled with possible emotional pain resurgence, might result in avoidance, creating voids where intimacy thrived. These challenges are common. Announcing them is the initial step toward recovery.

Rebuilding physical intimacy is a gentle and patient endeavor. A tenderness where honoring boundaries and comfort levels is insistent. Begin with non-sexual touches, emphasizing simple gestures like holding hands or gentle embraces. These actions take on safety and security, laying a foundation for deeper intimacy. Open communication is urgent in this process, encouraging candid discussions about desires and limits. Dialogues about suitability and restrictions open connected sensing and respect, allowing intimacy to unfold in its own time. Perceiving this as a unique inclination, accept that there's no rush or standard timetable for physical or emotional closeness.

Having a stake in emotional intimacy is equally important in the quest for reconnection. These silent moments strengthen a bond that transcends words, deepening emotional ties. Reinstating "date nights" as another tool allows for focused attention beyond grief. Whether through culinary exploration or simple home rituals, these acts celebrate enduring love beyond adversity.

Taking steps toward renewed intimacy requires persistence and empathy. This resurgence unfolds gradually, evolving at its own pace. Offer grace and give space for healing, both individually and as a couple, celebrating each small breakthrough along the way. Recognize minor victories without dismissing their importance, as progress fluctuates. Trust not only individual growth but also collective strength reflected in compassion and endurance. This route back to intimacy may reveal unexpected emotional hurdles, heightening the need for self and shared compassion. Healing is arbitrary, and it involves both strides forward and temporary setbacks. Some days will inevitably be simpler than others. Embrace these fluctuations and realize they don't define your relationship or its healing track.

Sustained communication is key as you rekindle both physical and emotional unions. Express any hesitations or worries transparently, emboldening interdependent trust and reaffirming your bond with your partner. Exploring new activities or experiences, unrelated to memories, supports intimate growth. Whether it's diving into fresh hobbies or joyful escapades, you spawn new memories devoid of loss. These serve as discreet advancements towards future joy filled expressions, testing a commitment to ongoing renewal.

In the revival of intimacy after miscarriage, revisit the truths underlying enduring, resilient bonds. Love transforms yet remains steadfast through rough circumstances, a reminder of strength against adversity, perseverance, and growth. Appreciate personal courage discovered individually and together. These are central qualities sustaining connection and underpinning long lasting love and healing.

Actionable Item: Intimacy Reflection Journal

Create an intimacy reflection journal to document small victories in reconnecting emotionally and physically. Note any activities that have invigorated your bond or challenges that arose. Tracking these will help visualize progression and inform future attempts to deepen intimacy.

FAMILY DYNAMICS: UNDERSTANDING AND SUPPORT

Miscarriage significantly reshapes family dynamics, causing subtle or sometimes dramatic shifts in roles and expectations. Families, typically a primary source of unity, might unintentionally add to stress through well intended advice or contrasting emotions. It's common for family members to offer guidance rooted in care and concern, yet these attempts can occasionally feel overwhelming. Such exchanges might breed frustration or isolation, magnifying the emotional weight already carried.

Managing these relationships calls for sensitivity, open communication, and ensuring family involvement remains supportive, not intrusive. Involving families in the healing process transforms burdensome interactions into constructive ones. Moreover, expanding the family's understanding of what truly aids in your healing expands their cooperation. Offering resources or articles that detail your experience can empower them with insights to enable compassion.

STRATEGIES FOR HEALTHY FAMILY INTERACTIONS

Develop lists of preferred family interactions that promote positivity and understanding. Encourage open discussions about grief's impacts on family interactivity and construct practical support systems that align with healing processes. Establishing boundaries within familial circles is monumental in protecting emotional health. Clearly conveying needs and limitations prevents possible tiffs. If specific topics cause distress, articulate these gently yet conclusively. Let family members know when certain discussions or events become overwhelming. This clarity aids in managing anticipations and reducing unintentional hurt. Establishing boundaries is not the same as exclusion; it propels a climate conducive to healing, devoid of additional tensions.

Promoting a supportive family environment encourages open, easy-going conversations about emotions and needs. Create spaces where everyone feels safe sharing without fear, enriching connection, thus strengthening bonds during unsettled periods. Family activities promoting unity, such as eating meals together or playing board games, offer continuity and togetherness, reasserting love as a central life force.

Families are inherently important to healing in the days, weeks, and months following a miscarriage. By involving them meaningfully and with well-defined boundaries, they bolster resounding support throughout recovery. Empower graciousness within familial ranks, turning potential pressures into strengths. Each interaction serves as a spotlight of vulnerability, growth, and healing. Through intention, these familial roles nourish indispensable networks, restoring stability in the middle of challenging times.

In wrapping up this chapter on managing relationships after a loss, we can agree that every interaction offers promise, a conducive way for healing. Relationships tested thus unveil grand opportunities for deeper growth. By intentionally shaping these compelling roles within your relationships, you receive a network of support that strengthens and uplifts.

Actionable Item: Managing Complex Family Dynamics

Craft a reflection on these interactions, exploring your feelings and responses to different scenarios involving pregnant friends and family. Encapsulate what aspects you handled well and areas where you might seek support in the future. This can serve as a learning tool for managing these inevitable circumstances.

CHAPTER 7
EMBRACING HOPE AND MOVING FORWARD

CULTIVATING HOPE: PRACTICES TO STRENGTHEN A POSITIVE OUTLOOK

THERE INDEED IS hope after a miscarriage, and it plays a role in the recovery process. Hope is a dynamic and evolving concept. There are practices that you can do to cultivate and sustain it. It begins with coming clean about your feelings surrounding grief and allowing yourself to feel every emotion that comes up. Seeking support and regularly engaging in self-care practices, such as getting enough rest and managing stress, can help your mental frame of mind.

Be kind to yourself by realizing that this process takes time, and consider professional help if you become overwhelmed by trying to do this alone. Professionals are armed with strategies to give you at the ready so you can minimize stressful thoughts. They can help you see that many miscarriage survivors can and do eventually have viable pregnancies. Choose your way to honor your baby's memory so that you can have peace and establish an informal relationship with other families in your situation to build up that sense of community and validation. Once this is achieved, you can start becoming more present during activities that you find enjoyable.

REDEFINING YOUR FUTURE: LIFE AFTER LOSS

Imagine a wide outdoor open space, a field representing your life's journey, dotted with the vivid colors of wildflowers dancing softly in the wind. Each blossom signifies a moment in your life's story, ranging from joy to sorrow, growth to struggle. It is within this expansive field that you find the opportunity to redefine how you perceive your future, especially after experiencing the deep impact of a miscarriage. While this loss is undeniably painful, it opens a portal for reflection and self-discovery, allowing you to become more attuned to your needs and desires. Through the lens of adversity, you might recognize newfound strength budding within you to explore the deepening of connections with others in powerful, unprecedented ways.

Reflect upon how your priorities have been reshaped in light of the loss. A reevaluation of your values can lead to empowerment and authenticity, guiding you towards a life fueled not solely by what was lost, but by what has been gained. As you embrace change, allow this metamorphosis to be a testament to your inherent strength and newfound perception.

Acceptance is critical as life looks different post-miscarriage, and this is where you can pivot yourself to discover peace and proceed with a new mindset. The concept of a 'new normal' is about declaring that healing is continuous, and expectations once held may require gentle realignment. View this transformation not as a deprivation but as an opportunity to harness change as a catalyst for growth.

CHARTING YOUR DREAMS AND ASPIRATIONS

Visualizing future aspirations is an empowering practice, reclaiming agency over the unfolding life before you. In envisioning the future, consider crafting a vision board that will be used as a tangible roadmap to encapsulate post-loss aspirations. Entwine images, words, and symbols reflective of the life you wish to embrace. This mosaic of dreams becomes a daily reminder, urging you towards goals with renewed bravery.

Different visual tools, like digital goal tracking apps, can be integrated into this process, offering structure and community support. Applications designed for setting and pursuing goals reinforce accountability and encouragement, developing a case towards personal growth. As you advance towards your dreams, these platforms become partners in transforming aspirations into reality.

Use this exercise to dream boldly, painting a picture of potential. This action inspires personal agency and encourages a purposeful stride into a future ripe with possibilities. By visualizing your goals, you're actively intertwining the aspirations into the fabric of your reality, fueling ambition along the way.

CREATING A NEW NORMAL: EMBRACING CHANGE

Transitioning to a new phase is a transcendent process of recognizing and commemorating each inflection point in your life. This period is not about erasing the past but integrating the lessons learned and the strength acquired into your current existence. Resilience becomes a staunch companion, teaching that growth is celebrated not only in powerful escalations of progress but also in gracious acceptance of life's unpredictability.

While we do not have the authority to change events of the past, we can use these major event markers to become agents of change. Change is hard, often because it lands you in unfamiliar territory. Seize the opportunity to create a new normal by choosing to accept what has happened. Making this choice in no way invalidates or minimizes your experience. A piece of you is forever lost, but that doesn't have to define your existence. Familiarize yourself with ways to honor your loss and remember that you don't have to physically perform an honoring task daily. You will become a stronger, more empathetic person once you complete the stages of grief. Someday, you may have firsthand knowledge of how to help someone going through this exact kind of trauma, and you will be healed enough to provide support without falling into the pits of sorrow.

ESTABLISHING RITUALS FOR STABILITY AND GROWTH

Crafting new routines instills a sense of foundation and balance. Consider initiating your mornings with gentle rituals, like taking a few contemplative moments before breakfast. Allow this time for gratitude and reflection to set the tone for your day. Evening routines of reading or meditative practices can offer closure, bringing a sense of tranquility before nightfall.

Acceptance of life's inherent unpredictability is a must-have for this process. Embrace that change is constant, and adaptation enriches life through unexpected beauty. Practicing mindfulness anchors you in the present, embracing the now while accepting the unpredictability of the future. This practice is all about a sense of calm, empowering mental clarity that propels you through life's ebb and flow.

Self-care is an intimate dance with the soul and body, incorporating small daily acts dedicated to making you feel good. Whether through exercise, nutritious meals, or opportunities to engage in creative pursuits, these practices beget growth. Each moment of joy adds a brushstroke of natural color to the canvas of your life, enhancing your existence with vibrant hues of happiness.

EMBRACING PERSONAL REINVENTION

The fearless pursuit of personal reinvention explores uncharted domains and discovers hidden parts of oneself. Whether it involves pursuing new interests, exploring potential academic advancements, or even changing careers, discovery refines self-knowledge. Ask yourself what you have learned throughout this process. Be sure to let go of old expectations by grieving the version of life you thought you would have had. Let go of that feeling of returning to how things used to be so that you leave the door open for growth. Your priorities may have shifted, so tap into that. Be empowered by your own voice and surround yourself with the kind of energy that can move you forward.

As life presents unforeseen opportunities, embrace them with exploration and wisdom. Remember, adaptability enriches your life. Personal evolution demands courage, patience, and an unyielding belief in one's capacity to surmount challenges. Seek the courage to overcome obstacles, celebrate triumphs, and frame fellowships with those who reflect your desires and aspirations. This will not only redefine you but amplify the horizons of your existence.

RECOGNIZING PERSONAL GROWTH

Personal growth is something you will be able to see if you are in tune with yourself. Look back at your reactions to certain situations versus the outcome. Zeroing in on how you respond can highlight your growth. Reflect on recent situations where you experienced something triggering or had an awkward moment with someone in public. Did you use self-compassion style language? Did you take a moment to choose another option before spiraling into old negative patterns? Are you more comfortable handling tough situations? Are you finding that you are letting go of blaming yourself and endless speculation? Hopefully, you can answer each question with a Yes. If not, that's ok too! This process takes time, and you may need more room to grow, so keep at it.

Track the small wins, because you'll need every ounce of positivity to get your jump start towards healing. If there was a day on which you found yourself having a good time, document it with the date and a brief description. If you held a boundary with someone who tried to pry for more information, document that too. If you asked someone for help with something, yes, you guessed it, document it! Refer to this record periodically to see that you really are making progress. You will be able to see where you were emotionally days, weeks, and even months ago. You may be able to recognize that even the tone of your inner voice is more positive.

Every encounter with hardship chisels your core, often exposing long-dormant strengths. Facing challenges reveals extraordinary inner strengths, with qualities honed and firmed up through overcoming difficulties. Adopting a hopeful disposition helps expedite this process. It acts as a lodestar, inviting brighter tomorrows. Welcoming this type of intention invokes a mentality geared towards growth and fulfillment. Not every day will be filled with rainbows and smiles, but welcoming the idea that every day is a fresh start helps build up positivity and a chance to see your own growth.

THE POWER OF ADVOCACY: TURNING PAIN INTO PURPOSE

Explore advocacy opportunities in your area. You can channel your experience into advocacy work and find purpose in helping others. Volunteering with miscarriage support organizations is one way to start. A quick internet search should reveal some local results. Creating awareness and educating the public about miscarriage is also impactful. Organizing community events or workshops is a great way to offer support.

If you prefer to go the online route, start a new social media support group to focus on emotional healing from miscarriage. While there are many groups already existing, they do not all have the same focus, style, or take on the same tone. You could tailor your group to a specific part of grieving a loss, grieving multiple losses, or even how to move forward with pregnancy attempts post-loss. The options are plentiful and can be a valuable source of information and support. Advocacy is a powerful tool in personal healing and development. Don't underestimate what it can do for you.

DRAWING INSPIRATION FROM OTHERS

Stories of others pictorialize the collective potential for healing present in every life. These accounts evoke reflections along the way, distinct yet analogous in the sophisticated mesh of human experience. With each renewed step, honor your capacity for adapting to change, allowing these new viewpoints to guide and inspire.

In recognizing the potential for group and individual transformation, embrace the events alongside others, knowing your testimony is part of a larger picture embedded with strength. Miscarriage survivors are strong, and brave enough to speak about their stories with others. Selfless acts such as these must be cherished. Listen to their stories and hold tight to the inspiring message they deliver. Let it serve as verifiable proof that emotional healing from pregnancy loss can and will most certainly be achieved for every one of us.

Inspiration can come from even the simplest of sources. It could be a brief exchange in a hotel lobby with someone checking out, or even from a store clerk organizing products on a shelf. People engage in small talk everywhere, sometimes volunteering personal and private information to strangers. This type of oversharing could benefit you. They may randomly go into detail about their miscarriage experience, as something in the environment could trigger a memory. As you listen, take in the information and realize the power of leaning on someone. Draw inspiration from their trials out of depression and visualize yourself in optimal mental health and thriving.

SETTING NEW GOALS: PERSONAL AND FAMILY ASPIRATIONS

Establishing meaningful goals after a loss involves intro- spection and alignment with core values. Applying method- ologies such as the SMART framework translates aspirations into actionable, tangible steps, propagating clarity and accountability. In goal setting, SMART stands for Specific, Measurable, Achievable, Relevant, and Time- Bound.

Let's say you and your partner decide to pursue adoption. The two of you dedicate time to researching your options and find that this may be a viable outcome for growing your family. Let's examine how the SMART steps can be applied to this scenario.

- **Specific** - You want to adopt a child between the ages of a newborn and 1 year.
- **Measurable** - You apply to an adoption agency and learn that four children fall into your preferred age category.
- **Achievable** - You and your family comply with all the prerequisite background checks to ensure a safe environment for the child.
- **Relevant** - You create a dedicated space in your home for the child to occupy, such as a nursery, and associated childproofing throughout the home.
- **Time-Bound** - You set a date by which it may be time to explore other avenues. Adoption can be a lengthy legal process that may take a few years to complete.

Don't be afraid to set a longer date to see the process through.

Goals resonate with a unique symphony of values that are all life's petitions to the heart, frequently involving family, career, and community. Embedded within familial dialogue lies the potential for unified visions and pursuits, where collaborative settings inspire mutual support and growth. Recognize that these aspirations are not solitary pursuits but intertwine deeply with those you hold dear. The collective movement towards achieving these goals strengthens bonds and transmits a supportive foundation to build the future.

OVERCOMING OBSTACLES TOGETHER

Overcoming challenges involves constructing strategies to circumvent obstacles and building a roadmap that can navigate the detours of setbacks. Engage those who inspire and guide you, such as mentors and role models, to expound on unfamiliar landscapes. Their wisdom provides a ladder to ascend, strengthened by experience and ready with solutions. Lean into this support system as often as possible, especially during periods of heightened emotions. Isolation doesn't have to be the answer. Oftentimes, it reinforces negative thoughts, which are counterproductive to your emotional well-being.

Maintaining an environment that encourages open dialogue and paired thinking is of the essence. It ensures stability and resistance. When faced with obstacles, you may lack the mental clarity needed to find effective ways to conquer them. For instance, if your kitchen sink starts backing up with water and won't drain properly, and you can't quickly determine the issue, ask your partner to handle the problem. Allowing your partner to take the lead on certain things, even temporarily, could save you from mounds of frustration. Your partner may be able to quickly resolve the issue by fixing it on the spot or submitting a work order to have it repaired. That may seem like a small task, but if concentration is no longer in your wheelhouse, then it may be time to solicit assistance in tackling obstacles.

Miscarriage calls for resilience permeated by patience and self-compassion, regardless of whether it is personal or familial. Every step marks a victory; any perceived misstep is merely a recalibration. Know that over time, you will build up endurance to overcome obstacles, whether they present themselves in small or large form.

REAFFIRMING THE VALUE OF GOALS

In moments of wavering doubt, reconnect with the foundational pulse, the core values of your aspirations. This reflection reignites determination, a passionate reminder of why these goals matter. Reaffirming the value of goals after such a deep loss is a nuanced yet achievable concept. You don't need to rush into productivity or achieve a goal right away, so do it when you feel the time is right. Start small by asking yourself what is needed to make you feel okay just for today. Don't worry about looking too far ahead, just move at a pace that starts out looking at short term goals.

Revisit your goals with compassion by asking why the goals originally mattered, and whether they still align in the aftermath of this experience. In doing so, you will reconnect to the reason behind your goal, even if the form changes. For example, the obvious goal may have been to start a family, but the deeper "why" could be to become a caregiver. This type of scenario is still feasible, although the process of getting there may differ from what was envisioned.

Feel free to create a short timeline of small steps to show intention. You could have a goal to write a one paragraph journal entry within the next seven days, then revisit the goal 30 days later to see how you feel. Allow your goals to shift as they are not set in stone, and engage in activities that still feel meaningful. Helping others can be masked as a distraction while providing healing and a sense of needed connection. Join hands with those who uplift you, sharing in thriving moments and tribulations, ensuring you are supported by those eager to walk beside you. Encouragement and practical support can transform challenges into triumphs.

Actionable Item: A Letter to a New You

Compose a letter to yourself, reinforcing the face of growth. In it, celebrate the ways in which you moved from lows to highs. These moments of self-reflection uplift your spirit, showing your strength. Be sure to cover your personal aspirations and how your support squad aided you in walking through one of the most treacherous times in your life. Mention how you overcame even a tiny obstacle and end the letter on a positive note.

CHAPTER 8
IT GETS BETTER FROM THIS POINT ON

FINDING JOY AGAIN: RECLAIMING HAPPINESS

REDISCOVERING happiness is a joyful chase imprinted with wonder and transformation. Revel in activities that bring joy—one where laughter flows freely, untethered by sorrow. Starting small with activities that you have previously enjoyed is a great way to reconnect with happier times. For example, something as simple as bird watching from your backyard could trigger memories from happier times. Get a small bird feeder and fill it with birdseed, then watch the show come to you. Set up a cozy seating arrangement in view of the birdfeeder, maybe even with a chair for another person. Ensure the seats are far enough away but still in view, so the birds do not hesitate to visit.

A change of scenery is always a great way to reset your mental health. Consider a staycation, if you will. You can book a hotel room in the same area where you live and stay there for two days. It doesn't need to be anything extravagant. The new-to-you setting can allow you to clear your head and not fall back into old patterns. If you have the means to travel further, consider booking a slightly further destination and visiting a place you have never been to. Be wary of guilty feelings for seeking out moments of happiness. Instead, frame it in your head as a reset towards restoring mental clarity.

Introduce some pampering into your routine to reclaim happiness. Designate a week in which you have one pampering activity a day scheduled for yourself. This will require some advanced planning, but it can be done. You could follow a schedule such as the one listed here:

- **Sunday** - Book a professional postpartum massage. Communicate with your massage therapist that you recently endured a miscarriage, and they will target specific areas of your body with a lighter touch.
- **Monday** - Treat yourself to a manicure and pedicure. You could have these services performed in a nail salon, or if you prefer, do it at home by yourself. If you choose the at home method, buy a new bottle of nail polish and perhaps select a color you wouldn't normally choose.
- **Tuesday** - Book an appointment at a hair salon for a basic service. It could be as simple as a wash and style, or if you want to go all out, you could add a cut and color.
- **Wednesday** - Apply a hydrating and soothing facial mask. Hundreds of facial products are on the market, so choose one that speaks to you.
- **Thursday** - Set the mood of relaxation by lighting scented candles. Aromatherapy in a relaxing environment can lighten your mood.

- **Friday** - Buy yourself a small gift. It could be an inexpensive bouquet of flowers, a new pair of sunglasses, a new phone case, or anything small that might bring you joy. There is power in retail therapy.
- **Saturday** - Get your body in motion by going for a leisurely walk. There are so many places to walk. It could be in your neighborhood, on the track at a local school, in a local park among nature, or even an outdoor mall.

ENGAGING WITH COMMUNITY FOR SHARED JOY

The pursuit of communal happiness roots itself in shared endeavors, and engagement creates threads between lives. The bonds conceived within these mutualisms season the spirit, granting strength to weather life's other challenges. Root joy in gratitude and shine a light on blessings. Engage in gratitude practices and allow positivity to infuse life's moments, accentuating a narrative where sorrow and joy coexist harmoniously.

Find joy in the small, everyday moments that bring content-ment and fully engage with each experience, highlighting the value in the ordinary and the extraordinary. Engage within communities in spaces where shared joy becomes an impactful vessel of connection and healing. Connect through mutual interests, volunteer efforts, or communal activities that bring jubilation. Recognize that in sharing joy, you also receive it, creating a cycle of positivity that can uplift even the heaviest of hearts.

Your personal escapade toward reclaiming happiness is underpinned by both the innate toughness crafted within and the parallel ties that bind you to others. Allowing yourself to steep in isolation can result in social malnourishment. Eliminate this from your life by starting small through engagement with passersby in public. Brief interactions with others, and then moving on, is a way to start.

A real-life scenario could play out like this: You go outside to check your mailbox, and someone is walking their dog nearby. Give a compliment to the dog or the dog walker. People love compliments, and it makes them feel good. Sharing in the joy of a compliment can boost the spirits of both parties involved. Another scenario could take place at work. Someone could walk in wearing a vibrant color or have a new hairstyle. Compliment the person and feel the joy. Oftentimes, people will compliment you in return.

Our friendships and covenant partnerships can hold more value than the exchange of compliments with passersby. An activity like eating a meal together in a new location can create new memories. Backyard picnics are a great way to start. Sometimes the bustling movements of a restaurant can be unbearable if the crowd size is too large. Enjoy spending time with your friends and family, reminding yourself that you do not have to be a topic of discussion. You can direct the conversation towards some of the goals or positive things that have recently happened in their lives and bask in celebrating those accomplishments.

EMBRACING A PERSONAL JOURNEY

Your journey toward happiness is deeply personal, a distinct voyage into the essence of self-renewal. Trust in your instincts and desires, recognizing the latent joy knitting together the threads of sorrow. With each stride, embrace your capacity for healing, rediscovered joy, and infinite potential. It's not about erasing grief but inviting its companion, happiness, to dwell alongside it.

The loss of a pregnancy can reshape your outlook on a variety of things. Take your time discovering what works best for you. One size fits all solutions cease to exist when it comes to something as personal as this level of healing. Fully embrace the experience and you will undoubtedly gain knowledge and become resourceful on this topic. Wherever you are in the healing journey is not the end all be all.

COMMUNITY AND BELONGING: SHARING SPACE WITH OTHER MISCARRIAGE SURVIVORS

The nature of the miscarriage survivor encapsulates an indomitable spirit, birthed not from invulnerability but from tenacity in the heart's vulnerable chambers. Participation in online forums and support networks reminds you of this power while you are within the designated space of strength and courage.

Immersing oneself within community initiatives serves as an expression of healing, offering others a lifeline while producing inner empowerment, all the while transforming personal experiences into opportunities for symbiotic growth. Finding a community with those who have a common history imparts understanding. Engaging in dialogues within these supportive spaces tells of lived experiences, modeling relations where stories breathe life and healing blossoms. Here, you will be provided with the opportunity to learn about new perspectives and hear firsthand accounts of various stages of the healing process, further validating your own experience. A community of miscarriage survivors provides targeted insight not otherwise found elsewhere. Support can come from anywhere, but receiving support from this community is exceptionally special as the members safeguard the same bond.

The associated values, interests, and goals found among miscarriage survivors can take some of the sting away during troublesome times. A huge benefit of joining this community is that you will receive a level of insight like never before. No one here is an outsider. If the lack of understanding in your own support system is a challenge, joining this community may be an effective way to rectify it. Community members provide support to one another and, in turn, receive uplifted spirits to aid in the progression of the difficulties. Engaging in retreats or group activities kindles introspection, dialogue, and collaboration. A powerful sense of compassion and collective progress flourishes within these support networks. This unity brings about a merging of strengths and reciprocal experiences, which can help to develop confidence that the miscarriage does not have to consume you.

SHAPING YOUR PATH FORWARD

Moving forward following a miscarriage is a tender and powerful process. Your path forward can feel like parts have been erased, making moving without those missing pieces seem impossible. If steps are taken to rebuild, anything is possible. Redefining what moving forward looks like to you may not involve returning to normal. Instead, it may mean learning to have joy and sorrow simultaneously, or even saying no to things that don't feel right anymore. Miscarriage can aggressively shake your sense of self, but you may discover strength, resilience, and vulnerability inside yourself that you never knew existed.

Leaning into others who have their listening ears on without trying to fix your grief is a form of support that you may require. Consider how community and belonging might sculpt rejuvenation. Embrace the potential in unity, an ongoing commitment to exploration in bridging the gap from isolation to association. Your future may look different, but just know the experience doesn't diminish your being. You may be more conscious and have extra layers of emotion, but you can still make space for hope by taking one step at a time. Every step forward is a dance of courage, and a song full of up-tempo beats awaits you.

CONCLUSION

I have provided you with practical steps to take to achieve emotional healing after pregnancy loss. As a reminder, you can use your phone to journal thoughts, seek out support in the form of trusted friends and family, seek professional interventions such as CBT or DBT therapy, get a memorial tattoo, create a family ritual to honor your loss, get moving through daily walking and light exercise, and make healthy diet and lifestyle choices.

As we end our time together, let's reflect on where we have traveled. This book has been a heartfelt exploration of the emotional, physical, and universal intricacies surrounding miscarriage. From understanding the medical aspects of pregnancy loss to moving through grief and healing, our focus has been on creating a supportive environment for recovery. We took the plunge into the significance of emotional healing, the importance of physical recovery, and the power of community support. These elements are not just steps but material companions toward healing.

Throughout the chapters, we've discussed the emotional vortex that follows a miscarriage. The passage through grief is deeply personal and varies for everyone. We've explored ways to embrace these emotions, to cry when needed, and to seek solace in journaling, art, and mindfulness. We've examined how these practices allow you to process your feelings, offering clarity and a sense of peace to intervene in chaos. By welcoming and accepting your emotions, you pave the way for healing to begin.

Physically, we've talked about the body's remarkable ability to heal after loss. We've discussed the importance of nutrition, gentle exercise, and medical follow-ups in fostering recovery. These practices support your body's healing and contribute to your emotional well-being. By caring for your physical self, you honor the connection between body and mind, creating a holistic approach to recovery.

Community and support systems form the backbone of this affair. We've emphasized the role of partners, friends, and family in providing love and understanding. Open communication and setting boundaries are key to keeping these relationships going. Whether through professional help, support groups, or online communities, finding your tribe who truly understands can be a source of immense strength and comfort.

As you transition from one phase to another, remember the key takeaways. We will get through this together. Miscarriage is a shared experience that many have faced and emerged from with newfound strength. Healing has many variables, and there is no right or wrong way to grieve. Your path is uniquely yours, and it deserves respect and compassion. By embracing your emotions, caring for your body, and seeking support, you create a foundation for healing and renewal.

I encourage you to take proactive steps in your quest to obtain healing. Reach out to those who can support you, whether they are friends, family, or professionals. Engage in practices that bring you peace and allow yourself the grace to heal at your own pace. Your strength lies in your ability to move forward, even when clarity is absent. The intense emotions that cover your being are only temporary. You may not see it now, but the deep sorrow and grief doesn't last forever. You may always have sad feelings about the situation, but it will no longer consume you one day. Getting over it is not the goal. Being able to accept, process, and cope with the trauma so that you can heal is where the finish line is.

I am deeply grateful to you for allowing my experiences to guide you. Your trust in this book and my journey is humbling. I want to reassure you that you have a place here. Healing is possible, and there is light beyond the darkness of loss. You have what it takes to overcome this sadness, and you deserve the compassion and understanding that comes from sharing your struggles.

In closing, hold on to hope. Hope is the thread that binds us to the future, offering the promise of joy and growth. Allow this to become a testament to your strength and courage. As you move forward, carry with you the knowledge that you can weather any storm. Embrace the possibilities ahead with an open heart and a spirit of resilience. Together, we have seen it through, and we are now equipped with tools to help others floating along in the same boat.

REFERENCES

- Miscarriage - Symptoms and causes. (2025). *mayoclinic.org*. Retrieved from https://www.mayoclinic.org/diseases-conditions/pregnancy-loss-miscarriage/symptoms-causes/syc-20354298
- Miscarriage - Afterwards - NHS. (2025). *nhs.uk*. Retrieved from https://www.nhs.uk/conditions/miscarriage/afterwards/#:~:text=Your%20partner%20may%20also%20be,can%20lead%20to%20relationship%20problems.
- The Effects of Stigmatized Grief. (2025). *cheservices.com*. Retrieved from https://www.cheservices.com/blog/the-effects-of-stigmatized-grief
- Miscarriage - Diagnosis and treatment. (2025). *mayoclinic.org*. Retrieved from https://www.mayoclinic.org/diseases-conditions/pregnancy-loss-miscarriage/diagnosis-treatment/drc-20354304
- Pregnancy loss: Consequences for mental health - PMC. (2025). *pmc.ncbi.nlm.nih.gov*. Retrieved from https://pmc.ncbi.nlm.nih.gov/articles/PMC9937061/
- 25 Grief Journal Prompts & Tips For Getting Started. (2025). *choosingtherapy.com*. Retrieved from https://www.choosingtherapy.com/grief-journaling/
- Mindfulness for Grief and Loss. (2025). *mindful.org*. Retrieved from https://www.mindful.org/mindfulness-for-grief-and-loss/
- Pregnancy loss support groups. (2025). *miscarriageassociation.org.uk*. Retrieved from https://www.miscarriageassociation.org.uk/how-we-help/support-groups/
- Physical Recovery After Miscarriage. (2025). *americanpregnancy.org*. Retrieved from https://americanpregnancy.org/getting-pregnant/pregnancy-loss/physical-recovery-after-miscarriage/#:~:text=Light%20bleeding%2C%20or%20spotting.,supportive%20bra%20may%20relieve%20discomfort.
- Nourishing Your Body After Miscarriage. (2025). *thefooddoula.com*. Retrieved from https://www.thefooddoula.com/blog/nourishing-your-body-after-miscarriage
- Exercises and advice following the loss of your baby. (2025). *royalberkshire.nhs.uk*. Retrieved from https://www.royalberkshire.

nhs.uk/media/x4zd5sj3/physio-exercise-advice-following-loss-of-your-baby.pdf

- Holistic Options for Miscarriage Management. (2025). *pinkelephants.org.au*. Retrieved from https://www.pinkelephants.org.au/page/86/holistic-options

- 6 Ultimate Ways To Create A Miscarriage Support System Now. (2025). *shrine-dev-node02.catalyst.harvard.edu*. Retrieved from https://shrine-dev-node02.catalyst.harvard.edu/6-ultimate-ways-to-create-a-miscarriage-support-system-now

- Coping with Loss Together: Strategies for Grieving as a ... (2025). *marriagefamilyservices.com*. Retrieved from https://www.marriagefamilyservices.com/post/strategies-for-grieving-as-a-couple/

- Emotional Healing After a Miscarriage: A Guide for Women ... (2025). *online.nursing.georgetown.edu*. Retrieved from https://online.nursing.georgetown.edu/blog/emotional-healing-after-miscarriage-guide-women-partners-family-friends/

- Online support: forum, email helpline, Facebook groups. (2025). *miscarriageassociation.org.uk*. Retrieved from https://www.miscarriageassociation.org.uk/how-we-help/online-support/

- After a Miscarriage: Surviving Emotionally. (2025). *americanpregnancy.org*. Retrieved from https://americanpregnancy.org/getting-pregnant/pregnancy-loss/miscarriage-surviving-emotionally/

- Talking to children about miscarriage. (2025). *tommys.org*. Retrieved from https://www.tommys.org/baby-loss-support/miscarriage-information-and-support/miscarriage-support/talking-to-children-about-miscarriage

- Supporting dads and partners through miscarriage. (2025). *tommys.org*. Retrieved from https://www.tommys.org/baby-loss-support/dads-and-partners/miscarriage-support

- Your Relationship With Your Partner After a Miscarriage. (2025). *tommys.org*. Retrieved from https://www.tommys.org/baby-loss-support/miscarriage-information-and-support/miscarriage-support/your-relationship-your-partner-after-miscarriage#:~:text=Communication%20can%20be%20hard%20when,about%20the%20baby%20we%20lost'.

- Supporting an employee before, during and after a loss. (2025). *miscarriageassociation.org.uk*. Retrieved from https://www.miscarriageassociation.org.uk/miscarriage-and-the-workplace/

employers-and-managers-information-and-support/supporting-an-employee-before-during-and-after-a-loss/

- Why can intimacy be so difficult after perinatal loss? (2025). *womenandbirth.org*. Retrieved from https://www.womenandbirth. org/article/S1871-5192(22)00347-X/fulltext

- How to Cope After Miscarriage. (2025). *nm.org*. Retrieved from https://www.nm.org/healthbeat/healthy-tips/emotional-health/ how-to-cope-after-miscarriage

- Rachel's story - The Miscarriage Association. (2025). *miscarriageassociation.org.uk*. Retrieved from https://www.miscarriageassociation. org.uk/story/rachels-story/

- Miscarriage & Early Pregnancy Loss Support Group. (2025). *emptyarmsbereavement.org*. Retrieved from https://www. emptyarmsbereavement.org/miscarriage-support-group

- A new look at the five stages of grief. (2025). *inside.wfu.edu*. Retrieved from https://inside.wfu.edu/2011/03/a-new-look-at-the-five-stages-of-grief

- 7 Obstacles that can stop us from asking for help. (2025). *the-haven.co*. Retrieved from https://the-haven.co/hard-asking-for-help/

- What's DBT? (2025). *dbtofsouthjersey.com*. Retrieved from https:// dbtofsouthjersey.com/whats-dbt/

- How to write SMART goals. (2025). *seek.com.au*. Retrieved from https://www.seek.com.au/career-advice/article/how-to-write-smart-goals